"*The Red Zone: A Love Story* is a period memoir as only Chloe Caldwell could write it, with warmth and particularity and charm. I smiled in recognition every few pages, read parts angrily aloud to my husband as though they were his fault, and laughed loudly enough at others to wake up my dogs. Yes, it's a love story, but *The Red Zone* is also an *adventure*, which may sound like a strange descriptor for a book about PMDD until you have experienced it through Caldwell's wry, piercing, fundamentally optimistic eyes. Both personal and communal, searching and exuberant, *The Red Zone* will speak to anyone who has been led by pain, curiosity, or misdiagnosis to become a detective of her own body."

—Kristi Coulter, author of *Nothing Good Can Come from This*

"The necessity and urgency of *The Red Zone* made me wonder how I—and any woman—had lived so long without it. Through the lens of PMDD and the female body, Caldwell refracts every issue imaginable, from relationships to hormones to queerness to stepmotherhood to blended families, all with hilarity, intimacy, and depth. Feeling seen by this book is an understatement; it's a survival guide."

—Zaina Arafat, author of *You Exist Too Much*

"A coming-of-age memoir for those of us in our thirties who are still trying to come of age, Chloe Caldwell's *The Red Zone* is an incredible tale of vulnerability, family, and periods. As hilarious as it is heartfelt, and as informative as it is inspirational, here is as honest a tale of self-discovery—and eventual self-acceptance—as has ever been written. A bloody brilliant book."

—Isaac Fitzgerald, author of *Dirtbag, Massachusetts*

"Finally (finally!) someone wrote a book about struggling to understand your body and your heart and finding the answers on the internet. This book is moving, funny, and impossible to put down. Caldwell reveals the messiness of life in a way few writers can pull off."

—Chelsea Martin, author of *Caca Dolce: Essays from a Lowbrow Life*

"Not since Elizabeth Wurtzel's *More, Now, Again* have I been so obsessed with a book of nonfiction. I read *The Red Zone* in one day, in one chair, four cups of coffee, and after: a single cigarette. Obsessed."

—Elizabeth Ellen, founder/editor of SF/LD Books and author of *Person/a* and *Her Lesser Work*

"Sentences like poetry, insights like medicine, the most romantic love story, the most spot-on depiction of life in the female body. I needed this book. Chloe Caldwell is among the most important literary voices of our time. Women are going to pass *The Red Zone* around forever."

—Diana Spechler, author of *Who by Fire* and *Skinny*

"*The Red Zone* is an intense, informative, highly entertaining book about the menstrual cycle, sexism, bickering, divorce, marriage, stepmotherhood, holistic gradual self-healing, and the layered effort to move from impulsivity and fear to stability and growth."   —Tao Lin, author of *Leave Society*

"*The Red Zone* showcases Chloe Caldwell at her best, with her trademark blend of humor and vulnerability. This is a special book, skillfully balancing practical knowledge and artistic deftness, and sharpness with sweetness."

—Juliet Escoria, author of *Juliet the Maniac*

PRAISE FOR

I'LL TELL YOU IN PERSON

"Caldwell is refreshingly regular and, German sojourn not-withstanding, unspoiled. Not once does the word 'internship' appear."   —*The Village Voice*

"Caldwell writes about her life with warmth, humor, and not a trace of apology."   —*Publishers Weekly*

"Her essays are diaristic in tone—they're unpretentious and personal and she draws powerful conclusions about what it means to grow into a decisive, fully formed person, if such a thing is even possible." —*HuffPost*

"The author's confessionalism has an engagingly conversational tone, yet the shock-value solipsism gives way to a stylistic maturity in which the author seems to develop command over her material." —*Kirkus Reviews*

"Caldwell's work is impressively devoid of horn-tooting. No humble-brags, no pity-parties. Just first-rate warts-and-all human complexity." —*Electric Literature*

"Unfortunately, when women write or speak about themselves with brutal honesty, everyone has an opinion. Conflating confession with universality, this literature is often dismissed for lacking inclusivity. It's as if society can only handle one woman—as long as she speaks on behalf of all women. Instead, we need more voices instead of asking women to speak for all women at all times." —*StarTribune*

"Caldwell makes it seem easy to speak with such a lively and intimate voice, but that's because she's a masterful writer. It's her deep and enduring compassion that gives Caldwell's essays both their literary and their moral backbone."

—*Heavy Feather Review*

"It will stay with you in its messy, funny, bitter, poignant, ecstatic, tragic wholeness while you read it and long after, as if it were a person you met at a party, one who you want to see again and again."   —*NYLON*

"Caldwell provides a pacing to her narrative which renders it impossible to put down; and, with a truth as fanciful as any fiction, there's no lack of plot twisting to drive each story home."
                                                      —*NewPages*

"Chloe Caldwell's sharp wit and keen powers of observation are in full force in her newest book."   —*PANK*

"Chloe Caldwell's *I'll Tell You in Person* is an intense collection of essays that astonishes with its self-awareness and keen storytelling."   —*Largehearted Boy*

"Chloe Caldwell is a force. A quirky writer who shares personal details of her life and describes them in a way that never feels like TMI, it's the opposite. You want more, the result of a trustworthy narrator and a skilled storyteller."
                                          —*Hippocampus Magazine*

"The job of the personal essayist is to make readers feel as if we know her. When she hurts, we hurt, as cohorts. When she wins, we win."   —*Vol. 1 Brooklyn*

PRAISE FOR WOMEN

"A writer like Caldwell doesn't need to follow elementary rules. Fanciful language would only distract from her narrator's candor, one of the book's greatest assets." —*The Barnes & Noble Review*

"Chloe Caldwell's slim and sensual new novella, *Women*, defies labels. It is not merely a love story, or a story of sexual awakening, or a coming out story, but a story about two women wrecking each other's lives during an illicit whirlwind romance."

—*Fjords*

"You might think a small-press autobiographical novella called *Women* that features one transgender man and texts with one cisgender man would find its way into the hands of only so many people. In the case of Chloe Caldwell's book, this has not been true. Perhaps because the story interacts with the reader, with The Narrator exposing her own fears, obsessions, and insecurities as we follow along." —*BuzzFeed News*

"The story is powerful [and] hot." —*Playboy*

"The book situates itself firmly in the precedent of queer women's fiction; hardly a few pages go by without a reference to Anne Carson, Jeanette Winterson, or, in one case, *The L Word*. Caldwell uses these as tethers for her own book, and earns a spot for herself among those she references. She brings to the page such an urgency that it is impossible not to be swept up, to remember what it was like when we ourselves were so engulfed by another person that when we emerged, we had to struggle to find ourselves again. *Women* is a skillfully and engrossingly written novella, a small slice of overwhelming love and heartbreak, and the search for belonging and self. Caldwell proves herself as a writer to watch in the coming years." —*The Masters Review*

"Chloe Caldwell's work is known for its vulnerability with her collection of essays *Legs Get Led Astray*. In *Women* we witness the narrator's recklessness, like when she throws her phone into the street with Finn on the line, or when she snorts coke that a date from OkCupid gave her, but we could also argue that it was the inclination towards recklessness and vulnerability that gave our narrator the possibility to explore this relationship and an identity that she hadn't considered before. It's reckless vulnerability that enables *Women* to take place."

—*Vol. 1 Brooklyn*

"Anyone who has suffered through apologetic fictionalized memoirs where the narrator spends every other page reminding you that she is 1) ashamed 2) confused 3) conflicted about the things that she is sharing with the reader will race through this nimble novella like a child gunning for the stairs." —*Fanzine*

"Nothing's sexier than first love and first intimacies, and Caldwell's brave autobiographical tale twists the trope into a powerful story about unexpectedly falling in love with a woman and the discoveries, sexual and otherwise, that ensue."

—*Time Out New York*

"What is refreshing about *Women* is its storytelling through the female gaze, and how this informs our questioning and resolution of identity. *Women* doesn't profess to be a feminist novella, and I didn't notice this distinction until I meditated on why the book feels so different from classic coming-of-age fiction and memoir."

—*Bustle*

"The keen eye and attention to detail made the book difficult to put down, and demanded that I read it in one sitting while also calling me to slow down and focus on the dust. Some of Caldwell's many strengths are in how she shows the intricacies, and dependencies, of relationships through an unflinching, unapologetic, and straightforward narrative."

—*American Microreviews and Interviews*

"The book is infused with savvy, dark humor, including a hilarious bout on OkCupid. Women at a queer dance party dress like characters from *Brokeback Mountain*; at a post-breakup coffee date, neither the narrator nor Finn will take off their sunglasses.

Hearts are broken, but Caldwell takes care of us. It's hard not to fall in love with this taut little book." —*Chronogram*

"What I love about Caldwell's writing is how it is satisfyingly disquieting in its relation to my own life. Selfishly, I wanted more. Not necessarily a tidier resolution—because how is life ever like that?—but I devoured the book in one sitting. I desired more exploration of these complicated feelings and the way we sabotage ourselves. The first time I ever fell in love, I didn't know it until she had already broken my heart. *Women* had me thinking about that and how first heartbreaks stick with us." —*Persephone* magazine

"*Women*, which is written in memoir style but is actually a work of fiction, is intimate and engaging from the first paragraph: The author explains that her pupils are expanding, which is either 'a symptom of falling in love or a side effect of the Chinese herbs my transgender friend Nathan was hooking me up with.' Perhaps it's the episodic structure and conversational tone that makes this 131-page novella easy to read in one sitting—or maybe it's just that good." —*Eugene Weekly*

"Caldwell has a directness and clarity in writing about herself that works really well, and the casual brushstrokes of her surroundings in a small, unnamed liberal city are precise. The transgender best friend, the coffee shop, the bars and library and house-sitting for wealthier friends serve to let the reader in rather than locking us out, harder to do than it appears to be."

—*An Anthology of Clouds*

"*Women* is a tiny novella, slim in page count and in circumference. You can, and should, read it in one sitting, so that it feels like stumbling across a friend's diary. It is packed with juicy details about the nameless narrator's relationships with the women in her life."

—*Bitch*

PRAISE FOR

LEGS GET LED ASTRAY

"For the reader, going astray means getting happily lost in the prose of Caldwell's daring, compelling, and graceful debut."

—*Publishers Weekly*

"*Legs Get Led Astray* swells with a bruised innocence and self-indulgence reminiscent of two great story collections that preceded it, Susan Minot's *Lust* and Mary Gaitskill's *Bad Behavior*. Like theirs, Caldwell's is a contemporary slice of sex and struggle."

—*Bitch*

"By exuberantly embracing her life, Caldwell invites the reader inside her emotions, experiences, memories, and reflections. She encourages the reader to enter her body. Her writing is a celebration of life, not a dissection. That difference is a relief. Caldwell lives without apology. It makes her collection stand apart from those that might be read as more traditional coming-of-age stories."   —*The Collagist*

"Caldwell's grasp on her own past, her ability to remove the lens of hindsight that sometimes fogs non-fiction, makes this collection one of the best I've read this year."   —*JMWW*

"The essays in this collection are as exuberant as they are sad. Her storytelling is as vulnerable as it is bombastic."
                                                        —*Rookie* magazine

"Ultimately, it's not Caldwell's specific experiences that generate this resonance in us, it's her precision of observing herself that allows us to turn the same microscope on ourselves. The same might be said of all effective memoir."   —*Metroland*

"*Legs Get Led Astray* is daring, funny, occasionally brilliant, and, above all, eminently readable."   —*The Faster Times*

"With work appearing on *The Nervous Breakdown* and *The Rumpus*, Caldwell's nonfiction reads like the bucket lists of a rebellious early-twenties indie darling. She writes about heroin hangovers and attending orgies. She's frank about her sexual exploits and masturbation tendencies. She captures an essence of trying to find her identity in an oasis of young bodies doing the same, testing mortality and making enough money for cheap rent and bodega Zebra cakes. Call it the haphazard lifestyle diet."

—Sabra Embury, *The L Magazine*

"A sort of 'autobiography as mixtape,' Chloe Caldwell's *Legs Get Led Astray* is a slim, 157-page book of personal essays that are brooding with sex and longing and repetition. It's also full of music, with B-sides like Elliott Smith, Nick Drake, Wilco, Rufus Wainwright, Tori Amos, and Okkervil River, whose lyrics in 'Last Love Song For Now' are where Caldwell's title comes from."

—*SF Weekly*

"This collection is hot and unpredictable: filled with the kind of energy that makes everyone envious. Attitude and presumption and wit."

—*Ringside Review*

"Her personal essays in *Legs Get Led Astray* lie in the same vein of feeling so intensely that it spills like filled rain gauges into your hands. She writes of so many normal things—lovers, brothers, children, camp, carrots, sex. But it is transporting; it is poetry. It is repetitions of magics in what happens to everyone, secrets that are so intensely and specifically personal that they are all of ours."

—*The Juvenilia*

"There's a density to the ways in which Chloe feels things. When the part of her that reads diaries she's not supposed to read and writes diaries she can't help but write meets the part of her that is reaching for truth beyond feeling, the results are deadly."   —*PANK*

"Annoyed as I was at times by how enamored Caldwell is with her own edginess, I was equally compelled by the way she relentlessly ferrets out the truths of her relationships."
                                                          —*Portland Mercury*

"Caldwell examines her relationships while she's still in the throes of them. Her essays talk about lovers, yes, but also about close friends, her parents, children she has cared for, and more than one instance of the Strand bookstore. Years of retrospect do not factor in here much—her feelings are still raw and maybe a little jumbled and maybe a little closer to the direct noise inside anyone's brain. Her heart swells and stretches, contracts and fractures, and her honesty is refreshing."
                                                          —*Persephone* magazine

THE RED ZONE

ALSO BY CHLOE CALDWELL

I'll Tell You in Person
Women
Legs Get Led Astray

THE RED ZONE

A Love Story

CHLOE CALDWELL

SOFT SKULL
NEW YORK

This is a work of nonfiction. However, some names and identifying details of individuals have been changed to protect their privacy, correspondence and PMDD episodes have been shortened for clarity, and dialogue has been reconstructed from memory, voice memos, emails, and texts.

For quoted material in the epigraphs, all reasonable efforts were made to contact the copyright holders.

Library of Congress Cataloging-in-Publication Data
Names: Caldwell, Chloe, author.
Title: The red zone : a love story / Chloe Caldwell.
Description: First Soft Skull edition. | New York : Soft Skull, 2022.
Identifiers: LCCN 2021037760 | ISBN 9781593766993 (paperback) |
ISBN 9781593767006 (ebook)
Subjects: GSAFD: Love stories.
Classification: LCC PS3603.A432 R43 2022 | DDC 813/.6—dc23
LC record available at https://lccn.loc.gov/2021037760

Cover design by www.houseofthought.io
Book design by Wah-Ming Chang

Published by Soft Skull Press
New York, NY
www.softskull.com

Printed in the United States of America
1 3 5 7 9 10 8 6 4 2

Dedicated to TK and LK

And for periods everywhere

By the time this is a book . . . this will all be resolved. Isn't that interesting?

EILEEN MYLES, *For Now*

Days ten and six and five before my period comes are the worst. The rest of the days aren't so good either.

SHEILA HETI, *Motherhood*

Statistics and newspapers tell me I am
  unhappy and dying.
That I need man and child to fulfill me.
That I'm more likely to get breast cancer.
And it's biology, it's my own fault.
It's divine punishment of the unruly.

JENNY HVAL, "That Battle Is Over,"
Apocalypse, girl

CONTENTS

PART ONE

FLUFFINESS

This morning we had a brief argument about my blood clots. Tony was making oatmeal and I asked if he would look at the photographs I took of my blood clots yesterday. I was feeling bold. I wanted to share the photos with someone, because they were so wild-looking. Chunky.

He told me he wanted to finish his oatmeal and peanut butter first. Then he'd look.

I got mad.

"If I was having a baby you wouldn't have the choice to eat your oatmeal first! There would be blood and guts everywhere!"

"I know the difference between having a baby and looking at a photograph! With a baby you don't have a choice. With looking at a photo, you do!"

I walked to my desk, laughing. I heard him muttering, "Jesus Christ," to which I thought, *Fair*.

He walked into my office twenty minutes later.

"Show me the blood," he demanded, like we were in a

Quentin Tarantino film, but I didn't want to. The urge had passed, and I wasn't proud of my blood clots anymore.

✦

According to my father, Tony was "like the best pianist in the world." A bartender had described him as a "crazy keyboardist."

He didn't look old enough to have a school-age daughter but when I first met him at my dad's music store in Hudson, New York, where I lived, there she was, bundled in snow boots and layers, power-clashing with stripes and polka dots. Tony wore ripped jeans and sneakers and a black hoodie. Later when I'd be in his life, I'd tell him to wear a coat. Then it was February and frigid.

That winter, I saw him once more; he was doing laundry, running back and forth from his car to his apartment, and I was doing exactly the same across the street at my dad's apartment. I thought it was funny that we were doing the same thing at the same time.

I did not see him for another year. I forgot about him. I led my single life. On Tinder, men's bios said they liked to *smoke meat* and *play guitar* and *drink whiskey* and *kayak*. On Tinder, men posed with alligators and crocodiles and beers. On Tinder dates, men's eyes glazed over while I spoke. Sometimes I played a game: seeing how long a date could go without the man asking me a question. Sometimes I went on dates with women, and they were better at asking questions.

One evening over burgers, a man explained he doesn't see the point of walking unless there's a destination spot like the cliff at the top of the hike. I walk almost every day with no destination, just aimless loops at land conservancies. I think, then, that the way we approach the outdoors can be deal breakers in relationships.

On a Tinder date, a guy said he didn't like a movie I like because it's plotless. "I like things without plot," I said. He ignored me. Told me what he knew about Scotch.

On a Tinder date, a man was "embarrassed for me" because I didn't know the filmmaker he was talking about. "Well what did he write?" I asked. "*Buffy the Vampire Slayer*," he said, looking at me like, *duh.* "Oh," I said. "Well then I'm embarrassed for *you!*"

He seemed offended when I said that. Why was it okay for him to say it to me but not me to him? He listed four more movies and shows the filmmaker had written.

"Oh. Well I don't like that genre," I told him, "so there's no way I would know that guy's name."

"It's actually five genres I just listed," he said.

"I don't like any of them."

I took the trash out. Did the dishes. Wrote books. Girlfriends, girlfriends, girlfriends made up my life. More Tinder.

Netflix. Humble book tours. Airplanes. Airport bars. Amtrak trains. Girlfriends. Wine with my mom. Trips with my mom every April. Friends from middle school; friends I'd just made at readings. At twenty-nine and thirty, I still had sleepovers. Women slept on my futon. I slept on women's floors in Crown Heights and Clinton Hill. Women were my plus-ones to everything. We rented bunk beds at the Jane Hotel. We did one another's eyebrow makeup. Flew in for one another's birthdays. There was never a shortage of women to experience life with. A friend gave me a patch that read EMBRACE PLATONIC INTIMACY.

When these women, my friends, began to pair up around age thirty, I had to suppress the abandonment I felt. I smiled with my teeth, and was happy for them in my heart, but it wasn't without a sense of panic. I accepted that I'd become married to writing, go to literary parties, have flings. My career seemed like it was going well. I didn't have any money, but I was in some magazines and a good number of celebrities were Instagramming my books, and it didn't get much better than that, right? I'd been introduced at a wedding as "single as the day is long." I'd been included in an article in *Elle* magazine, published for Valentine's Day, called "41 Hottest Singles of 2017." *We have curated a list of the most eligible and fascinating single people to be around, and you're one of them*, the email read, and invited me to New York City for a photo shoot.

Single was becoming my brand, my identity. Some days

it almost felt like something to be proud of. There was a new genre of books about being single. I bought them all, though I only read parts: *Spinster: Making A Life of One's Own*; *All the Single Ladies*; *It's Not You: 27 (Wrong) Reasons You're Single*. The books lay around my room, my bed, my coffee table. I posted them to Instagram. Skimmed through them without fully committing.

There was a certain route to the nature trails I walked on outside of town, where I'd drive by purple signs with white font that read: APPLY FOR A FOSTER CHILD TODAY. Whenever I saw one, I became curious. I'd always wanted a child in my life. I'd loved the challenge of connecting with children, whether these children were my friends' kids, kids I babysat, kids I met in restaurants. I was interested in non-blood bonds. I remember having brunch with my friend Karina, a bit hungover during a book tour, and out of the blue telling her I was planning to adopt a kid at age thirty-five if I hadn't met anyone by then. I remember her slight surprise at my non sequitur. I'd thought that if I said it out loud, I'd actually do it. Thirty-five seemed light-years away; I could dump ideas and lifestyles on it because it was so abstract.

Most days, I felt energized about my unconventional life. I was the female role model I'd always needed. Some women needed to stay single to show the younger generation it could be done. That you could live alone, be financially stable, have your own career.

Not having someone to rely on was also stressful. About twice a year, when I was trying to take the bag out of the trash and I needed a second pair of hands to hold down the can as I pulled it out, I did want a partner. Or when my car was covered in four feet of snow and wouldn't start.

"I am so *sick* of doing everything myself," I said to my roommate.

One evening when the temperature was below zero, I was attempting to unlock the door to my apartment while juggling grocery bags when my landlord opened it from the inside for me. "I heard struggle," she said.

She was right. Those days I had so little money, I'd often grocery shop at CVS. Eggs and toast can take you far when you're broke. When I'm home and not sure what to do with myself I boil eggs. Boiling eggs gives me a sense of control in a world of chaos. I even buy them at Penn Station, eat them on my trip home, sometimes with those sad little salt and pepper packets. I like how you can put eggs on to boil and go take a shower while they do. I like how it's something to do every day that is the same, but they always turn out a little bit different.

✦

What would it be like to have a partner who would encourage you to go to yoga? Or would they encourage you to stay home? I did not understand how partnerships worked. I did not comprehend their complexity; I thought they only inhibited you or encouraged you, with no middle ground.

When I was twenty-seven, a friend of mine told me: *I just want you to know,* she said, *you deserve someone who wants to sleep with you* and *make you eggs in the morning.*

Touched as I was by this sentiment, I was positive it would never happen to me. I was so loose in the world for so long.

I spent the majority of my coming-of-age with my divorced mother, and I remember one evening in the winter I was twenty-nine going to a film alone, eating popcorn alone, and having the acute feeling that I had the energy of a divorced woman. I felt I had been through a divorce myself. I suppose I had: my parents' divorce.

One winter when I was twenty-nine and at the movies, it clicked: I decided the only person right for me would be a divorced person with a child. I passed it off as a joke, to my therapist, to a few friends, to my mom. I thought it was a clever quip, but deep down I meant it. You aren't supposed to want someone divorced, with baggage. You're supposed to want someone who is a clean slate—but I didn't. I had a past, and as an author and essayist, my past could be known. Divorced people's pasts couldn't be hidden, either.

I kept talking about my friends' coupling up as though it were a disease. I skipped over the parts of people's essays where they wrote about their partners. Boring, boring, boring. Unrelatable.

I visited my nana with my mom, and one of my uncles was

there. We were admiring a handmade cutting board he'd made, and he said he gifted them to each of my cousins when they got married. I was vocal about wanting a cutting board, too.

He told me he wouldn't make me one unless I got married.

"What if I never get married?" I said.

I had no prospects. I was much more interested in writing books than I was in marriage. I mean, I didn't want a hand-made cutting board *that* bad.

"It happened to *Logan*," I told Karina.

"It happened to *Colleen*," I told Emily. I knew how silly this was—did I expect us all to stay single as some kind of unspoken solidarity? (Kind of!)

✦

On Amtrak to New York City at the end of March, for an event called "I Wrote a Book: Now What?" I was swiping Tinder—I was always half-heartedly swiping Tinder. *There is no one new around you,* Tinder would say. But I saw the best pianist in the world, the crazy keyboardist, was on Tinder; single again.

It was very low stakes; I only messaged him the word "Hey." He asked me if I wanted to go see music the next night. I asked him how his daughter was doing.

I wasn't sure I wanted to go on a date. God, I'd been on so many already. But when I arrived home from the city, a black dress I'd ordered had arrived. The tag said GLAMOROUS, and

I wanted to have a reason to wear the dress. In the bathroom, I put on what they call a panty liner, because it was the last day of my period and there wasn't enough blood for a tampon. It also assured me that I'd go home that night. I powdered over my acne, put on my brown boots.

We talked until 3:00 a.m. First standing across from each other in his kitchen—he stood in front of the stove and I stood in front of the counter.

"You ask questions," he observed at one point, holding eye contact. "You listen."

Other people don't? I wondered.

I liked his bathroom. I didn't know that twelve months later I'd be painting the walls of it teal, that my blood clots would be on its floor. That I'd be bleeding in the shower, trying to calm my cramps in the claw-foot tub. I didn't know his daughter, Sadie, would be asking me to make her baths.

She loved how much lavender bubble bath I'd pour in. Her blue eyes got wide. She called the baths "fluffy." "It's so *fluffy*!" she'd squeal, delighted. "Everything needs to be *fluffy* for me to like it! I love *fluffiness*!" Turned out I loved *fluffiness*, too; I'd just never had language for it before.

Drinking the seltzer he handed me, I sat on the floor by the bookshelf, under the guise of looking at his books. I didn't want to sit next to him on the couch. It felt too intimate. On the shelf I saw the book *Spiritual Divorce: Divorce as a Catalyst for an Extraordinary Life* and something in me settled.

When therapy came up, it was revealed we had the same therapist, Anna, and that we both had been going to her for three years. Later, he told me that when I found this out, I moved to the couch from where I'd been on the floor. He told Anna the same thing, and she told him that it was very observant of him to notice.

"It's like our lives had been going like this," he said, making figure eights with his hands.

It is mysterious—how we did not see each other at the post office, the bar where I loved my tequila cocktails and he loved boulevardiers. The laundromat where I usually did drop-off and where he spent his Sundays. The coffee shop where he always gets a large hot and I get iced.

When I walked home to my apartment at four in the morning, I counted how many steps it took. Four hundred and fifty-seven. Just under four minutes.

He told me he'd saved the tab on my seltzer can. I'd taken it off because since age ten I'd learned to pull it back and forth while going through the alphabet. The letter the opener breaks off on is the first letter of the last name of the person you're going to marry.

He'd gone around the house looking for the seltzer tab. I'd left it on the bookshelf. He put it in his pocket and sent a photo to me a few days later.

The second time we met for a drink, we played the Cheese Game, which my friend Noelle and I used to play at bars. On a napkin, you list all the cheeses you can in sixty seconds. Then you read your lists, crossing out the ones you both wrote. Whoever ends up with the most original cheeses wins. Tony, being from Wisconsin, seemed like the best person to play with, but I won the game with flying colors. Later, when I told Noelle, she kept saying, "I can't believe you guys played the *Cheese Game* together," as though I'd cheated on her.

A few days later when he showed up at my door with spring forsythias, shockingly yellow, I pretended everything was normal, that people rang my buzzer all the time to bring me flowers and notes. The flowers were so tall they hit the low ceiling of my apartment, which a friend said was like the apartment in *Being John Malkovich*.

"Forsythias for your first apartment living alone," he said.

My dad happened to be over. We were moving my furniture and having a hard time fitting a couch through the narrow doorway of the old apartment. I invited Tony inside and my dad asked him if he wanted to help us move the couch.

When he left, I texted him that yellow was my favorite color.

"Do you date him?" my dad asked about his neighbor.

I was embarrassed, downplayed it. "I went on one date with him. We have a lot in common."

"Oh yeah, definitely. He's like the best pianist in the world," he said again.

"Yeah, you told me."

◆

After only hanging out twice, Tony asked if I could go with him and Sadie to the airport, *and* pick them up a week later when they returned from Madison, Wisconsin, where they were going for Easter. I couldn't believe he was planning a week out. It seemed nuts.

We listened and sang along to *Hamilton* and the Beach Boys while we drove. I noticed Tony ate wintergreen Altoids like I did: as though they were a full meal. The weather was epic and I felt a surge of joy and relaxation I hadn't felt in a long time. I did not feel I was missing out on any other kinds of life experience, and it was surprisingly clear to me I was with the two people I was meant to be with. That day or forever? I didn't know. There was something so attractive about Tony's energy, his preparedness for this trip with his daughter, the way he'd braided her hair that morning and dressed her in unicorn leggings.

Tony and Sadie walked toward the airport, and Sadie yelled back to me, "See you on the twenty-first!"

I made a couple of stops on my drive back, just to sit in the sun or change the music or call friends. I stopped at the farm store with a sign that read EASTER PUSSY. It was supposed to say EASTER PUSSY WILLOWS, I think. In the store, I was suddenly noticing kid toys, candy for kids. I parked on my street when I arrived back in Hudson. How did I now have someone else's car, someone else's keys?

It was a big deal to be able to afford my own apartment. My mom had told me she'd never lived alone, and it was a regret of hers. At thirty-one, I'd never lived alone either, and I'd never lived with a partner; it was roommates and friends for the last decade. She came over when I was finished moving in, and we toasted with champagne. The afternoon sun was incredible.

✦

Tony tried to sleep over the night after he'd slept over for the first time. He was so natural, taking off his socks and T-shirt, as if it was something we'd done a million times before. But I wasn't ready for it.

"Don't take this the wrong way," I said, "but you can't sleep over again. It's too intimate for me."

"Okay," he said. "I'll walk home."

We sat at my oak table for another few hours, talking, laughing, drinking fernet. I explained I was too guarded to have someone sleep over two nights in a row. It meant too much. I was trying to be careful.

"I just want you to know that sleeping next to someone every night can be the opposite of that. It can be really grounding," he said.

Yeah right, I thought.

"What do you look for in relationships?"

"I don't," I said.

"I think there's something you're looking for," he said.

"Like what?"

"A connection."

"Maybe."

"Well I'd like to try being in a relationship with you."

I remember having, or trying, to cover up my smile and shock. No one had ever been so direct with their language, so present, so sure.

"That freaks me out, that you said that," I said.

◆

The first time I slept over at his apartment, I bled all over the sheets. An enormous pool of the brightest red. Tony was calm. "Menstrual blood isn't like other blood," he said, and cleaned the stain off efficiently. How did he know this, and I didn't? What made it different from other blood? I'd never thought about it, but if I had, I would have assumed the opposite. To me, menstrual blood always felt permanent.

Those first couple of months, I constantly forgot where I left my car, only to find it covered in red-and-white parking tickets. My keys were always lost; I stopped eating anything except fried chicken from the bar we went to late at night, yet ten pounds fell off my frame. Every day was a celebration. We read in front of the Hudson River; we bought picnic baskets. We listened repeatedly to "You're My Favorite Waste of Time" by Marshall Crenshaw. We were each other's waste of time, drinking fernet until three in the morning and then until one in the afternoon. In the mornings, we drank coffee with maple syrup, spending hours across from each other at the oak table, and then it was noon and we both had to get on with our lives. Sometimes when I glanced at the clock and saw a number, it'd take a second before I knew whether it was a.m. or p.m.

Almost always, there were fresh flowers in my kitchen, gifted to me for no reason at all.

He walked into the kitchen one morning and said, "I think you kick your socks off in your sleep."

"I go to bed with socks on and get hot at night. How'd you know?"

"I found twelve socks in the bed when I was making it."

Making the bed was something I half-assed. I'd half-heartedly throw the covers back up sometimes if people were coming over.

He told me when he was at the New England Conservatory, there had been a visiting lecture from a professor at Juilliard. The professor had warned the students that they'd be coming home from gigs or auditions dejected and exhausted and that a made bed was one small thing they could do for themselves. He continued to make my bed every single morning.

I liked that Tony had received a scholarship when he was fifteen, to Interlochen Center for the Arts, because, as a Jewel fan, I knew she too received financial support to attend

Interlochen. And though Jewel and Tony are seven years apart, secretly I pretended Jewel was his ex-girlfriend.

✦

"I wonder how this is going to end," I said aloud one night while we were lying next to each other in my bed.

"Why does it have to end?" he asked.

"Because everything ends," I said.

My apartment morphed from a bachelorette pad into Sadie's favorite place for hide-and-seek. The three of us watched *Freaky Friday* in my bed, and in the mornings we played hangman, I spy, and Legos. When Tony would ask me if I had something some people consider an essential kitchen item, like hot sauce or a bread knife, I'd stare at him blankly.

I used a space heater in my apartment, even in April and May. I was always cold. Tony used a fan in his bedroom. One night, Tony had an extra ticket to the comedian Steven Wright and invited me. I didn't want to go, too tired and burnt from all the late nights. Tony surprised me by inviting my dad to take my place. When he came to my apartment after the show, a little before midnight, I was already in bed. Influenced by Wright's deadpan humor, Tony began doing a bit about my space heater, which lived on a stool, because all of my stuff lived on stools: plants, decorations, and now the heater.

"Stop making fun of my space heater," I said.

"I'm not making fun of your space heater. I'm making fun of your stool."

✦

One perfect June afternoon, we bought dirty chais and walked to an old theater in town where the best pianist in the world would play for me for the first time. I sprawled on a couch; he wore a button-up shirt and played renditions of Radiohead, Aphex Twin, Vince Guaraldi Trio, and *West Side Story*. The caffeine made me more in love, if that was even possible. I felt clammy, dreamlike. The perspective of the town I'd live in for years had changed.

"I want to share life with you," he said, two months into dating. We were in the Catskills, drinking champagne, and I was smiling so big I was tempted to cover my mouth.

One morning when he left my apartment for his own, he saw I'd put a jade plant I'd killed out in the trash. When he got home, he texted me a photo of it on his windowsill. "I don't have the greenest thumb," he said. But he was trying.

For the entire next year, I found forsythia petals in cracks and corners whenever I swept.

SCUM BEACH

The beach on your period isn't impossible but I wouldn't exactly describe it as relaxing. In June, for the second year in a row, two girlfriends and I were driving to Branford, Connecticut, to stay at my friend's family's beach house on Scum Beach.

Noelle parked outside my apartment. I felt tired and cranky and anxious about a cyst on my cheek, which I did my best to pretend wasn't happening. (I had recently listened to the writer Melissa Broder on a podcast and she was talking about chin zits. She was explaining that as soon as she meets up with someone she'll be like, "Look at the chin zit, look at it." I sort of envy this, but it's not my style. She says it's a control thing, that she wants the person to know that *she knows* it is there. But my perspective is: I know it's there, my friend knows it's there, my friend knows I know it's there, and I don't feel like talking about it.) The cysts sometimes came once a month, sometimes once a season.

Earlier that morning, I'd gone to a yoga class. The room

was packed, and a tall man I'd never seen with curly hair and many tattoos put his mat directly in front of mine. It was a tight squeeze and his long legs and feet were almost touching my mat. The tattoo on his foot, facing me, read, in all caps: SCUM FUCK. This took my mood from a three to a ten.

◆

In middle school and high school, a friend whose locker was next to mine would ask me, as we fiddled with our locks each morning: "One to ten?" about where my mood was. One being horribly depressed and ten being high on life, as we called it then. I guess I've been tracking my moods ever since.

When I looked at my old diaries recently, specifically the first diary I kept at age eleven, I see that I rated my days. I think I copied this from the narrator of the Judy Blume book *It's Not the End of the World*. I kept at it for years: A-, C+, and B.

◆

Noelle drove my car and I rode passenger. When I'm taking trips with my friends, I am often so excited to be with them that I can't drive and talk at the same time; I lose focus on the driving part. We hadn't gotten very far when I needed to pee like crazy, so we stopped at a gas station.

I went into the grimy Stewart's bathroom and there was

blood. Accompanied by cramps. Followed by diarrhea. I began panic-popping ibuprofen, and over the next hour and a half we stopped four more times.

✦

Baffling: why, each month, do I rush to buy tampons and pads? Why, when—like death—getting my period is one of the only certainties in life, am I not prepared for it? It's the same with razors. Why do I have to rush and buy them each month when I know my leg hair will grow back?

According to "Here's How Much a Woman's Period Will Cost Her Over a Lifetime" in *HuffPost*, we are expected to use 9,120 tampons in a lifetime. "On average, [menstruating people have their] period for three to seven days and . . . menstruate from age thirteen until age fifty-one. That means the average [person] endures some 456 total periods over thirty-eight years, or roughly 2,280 days with our period—6.25 years of [their] life."

I imagine the 2,280 days are referring to bleeding. Seven days of PMS symptoms each month, the number is 3,192 days, or 8.7 years.

If you add 3,192 days of symptoms to 2,280 days of bleeding, the answer is 5,472 days. The unit converter website tells me it is: 14.9917 Years = 14 Years, 11 Months, 3 Weeks, 6 Days, 9 Hours, 16 Minutes, and 59 Seconds.

Tampons have always been off-putting to me. You're plugging yourself up when you're supposed to be flowing. Logically it just seems weird.

When I lived with my dad in my twenties, I'd often see a box of my cotton tampons on the dinner table. My dad used them for playing the hurdy-gurdy. I recently asked him about it:

"I shouldn't tell you because if it gets out it will ruin my reputation in the vielle à roue (hurdy-gurdy) community. I was told to get this special cotton that's really hard to find . . . I talked to a bunch of people at the gurdy festivals in France and Quebec about where to get it, etc. I was told regular cotton balls wouldn't work. I first used a tampon (I don't know whose it was but it had never been used) because there was no other cotton available.

"You have to cover the gurdy strings in cotton right where they rub against the wheel. Just a teeny bit. It takes a lot of practice. The wheel is turned very slowly and then I try to get the cotton (which is pulled gently into a half inch or so square) to twist around it. When the cotton goes under the wheel, I flick it with a finger so it rolls around the string like a sheath, grab and twist the string, and the cotton rolls around it, the string doesn't touch the wheel, just the cotton does. The cotton softens the sound."

That's my favorite way tampons are used.

◆

Two comedians I love, Catherine Cohen and Pat Regan, host a podcast called *Seek Treatment* and once they were saying there are two kinds of people in the world: those who feel small when they stand beside the ocean and those who feel normal-sized. I'm the latter. The ocean doesn't make me feel anything. (How many people did I just alienate? Definitely my mom.)

On my beach towel, my blood stained my vintage high-waisted light denim Levi's shorts. I'd splurged on them, and now blood had splurged on me.

On Instagram later that day I posted a photo Noelle took of me walking toward the ocean, in a borrowed blue bikini top and the Levi's shorts. I captioned it: *31-year-old with cramps of a sixteen-year-old.*

"That ain't right," my aunt commented.

"Take magnesium!" someone else said.

We went out for drinks and dinner that night at a hipster barbecue place and sat outside at a picnic table. Midmeal, I went to the bathroom feeling sick. I had blood clots coming out of me, and diarrhea. I had a headache and cramps and felt shaky. I stayed in there a while, crying and letting everything empty out of me.

I thought about a gynecologist I had a follow-up to a Pap smear with once. She asked me if I was okay because she saw me walking strangely coming into the office. I didn't look good, she'd said. I just have my period and am sick, I told her.

"Let's do something about that, why don't we?" she said,

going on to explain that the blood and diarrhea caused my serotonin to flush out of my body. This was why, she explained, some women went on antidepressants in the week leading up to their period through day three or so of bleeding. She was implying that I could, and should, be one of those women.

I ignored her and left my appointment.

I still don't know if she was right about that, but every time I have diarrhea now, I think of her. <3

Jen Gunter, writer of the *New York Times* women's health column The Cycle and author of *The Vagina Bible*, writes that "menstrual diarrhea is experienced by more than 25 percent of otherwise healthy people who menstruate." Yet it is rarely—if ever—discussed. Even in the doctor's office.

Back at the picnic table, I burst into tears telling my friends how sick I was. They softened. I asked them if they got this sick on their periods. Not really, they said, though Caroline said she became a "she-wolf" the days before her period. She'll go out and have a bender, a surge of energy, make poor decisions.

We walked back to the beach house and decided to watch the new *Beauty and the Beast*. We'd started the movie and were having some drinks when Tony called. I went outside to speak with him.

Tony mentioned that he'd gone on a hike and that two female friends were supposed to be there, but that he didn't end up running into them.

I paced around in circles. The details were blurry but the feeling was acute: I felt like he was lying to me. Fucking with me. There was no talking me down—I'd convinced myself Tony was an asshole, tricking me.

"Why do you want to get off the phone with me?"

"I don't think this is productive."

"Is there something I should know? Something you aren't telling me? Why does it feel like you hate me?"

Remember that Harvey Danger song from the nineties? *Paranoia, paranoia, everybody's coming to get me.* I loved that song. Now that line was my life.

Though I'd had PMS in my day, it was the first time I'd felt this way, ever. This was new.

That night, Noelle and I slept in bunk beds in the kid bedroom. The sheets were covered in princesses. Twice in the night I woke up to have ibuprofen, taking deep breaths, tossing and turning and asking my cramps to kindly stop, bargaining with them.

I remember one night in high school my cramps being so bad I slept in my mom's bed. They were so terrible that I named each one as they moved through me. I was delirious. I told my mom the next day and she didn't believe me. She said, *You were so out of it, I can't believe you'd be able to do that.* She told me that when she'd gone into labor, she was shocked to realize her labor pains were quite similar to the menstrual cramps she had had in her twenties.

In the morning, we walked to get coffee and breakfast sandwiches and I was feeling a little better.

We drove home during rush hour and were in traffic, at a standstill for hours. We found an old Lucinda Williams cassette tape in my car and listened to her songs from 1979, before she was famous.

Even now, four years later, Noelle remembers my period that month. "Something was wrong," she says now. "I felt bad for you. You were really sick."

When we arrived back in Hudson, Tony and I went to dinner. We sat at the bar of a French restaurant in town and spoke about the awful phone call. How it confused him. He explained it felt like the rug was pulled out from underneath him.

Something wasn't right. Since I'd gotten into my thirties, my periods had become more severe. Why was it heightened? Why was I afraid of it? It was affecting my relationships and my ability to socialize; it had ruined my weekend away. This didn't feel like just PMS. It felt different. Dangerous.

When I open a notebook from this time in 2017, I find this: *my moods are scaring me. Once a month I have these massive outbursts.*

I don't remember having PMS as an eleven- and twelve-year-old or as a teenager, though I must have and didn't have the word for it. Maybe it manifested in those fights with Mom, or as taking those three-hour after-school naps. Maybe it manifested as the big red zits I sometimes got on my otherwise calm skin. Maybe it manifested as the hot chocolates I loved getting at the gas station. Maybe it manifested as those days I was too depressed to go to school. Perhaps it was part of the reason I loved smoking weed as a teenager. It's certainly what many women use now for their cramps and moods. I've even been recommended THC suppositories by a woman at a THC shop in Colorado. But she told me they were so strong she couldn't walk, so I skipped purchasing them.

✦

How unfortunate that khakis were the popular pant during the years we were eleven, twelve, thirteen, fourteen. We'd walk around saying "Check my butt" to each other. Pads in our pockets, tampons in our lockers. The smell of blood—the way you can smell the blood before you even begin bleeding. Rusty. Why did we have to wear what everyone else was wearing? Why couldn't we have been empowered enough to change the trend—to wear dark denim? Or black? It had to be khakis from Old Navy or Gap, American Eagle or Limited Too.

On Instagram, an ad tells me to "say goodbye to leak anxiety," but without leak anxiety, who would I be? How many hours of my life have I spent wondering if I was bleeding through my pants, realizing I'd bled through my pants? How many pairs of jeans and underwear have I ruined because the blood came early or late, or more heavily than I'd anticipated?

Doctors and commercials and gynecologists and even friends often ask if your period is heavy. Articles and books and podcasts refer to heavy periods. If your period is "heavy," you might have a problem. But the *real* problem is that we were never told what a "regular" period should look like. At least in my middle school or high school, we were never handed three buckets of blood and told which one was light, regular, and heavy. We were never told how many tampons or pads was "normal" to fill during a period. I don't know if my period is heavy. I can only guess. Some months I bleed more than others. Heavy compared to what? Compared to whom?

In *Periods Gone Public: Taking A Stand For Menstrual Equity*, activist Jennifer Weiss-Wolff says that often when she told people she wanted to get tampons in schools, they'd say, "Tampons? What about condoms?" As if they are one and the same.

Sometimes I imagined photographing each bloody design I bled into the toilet for a year to see how different they were. Once I texted a particularly pretty image of my blood to my friend Karina.

"Mine doesn't spread out like that," she responded.

"Mine usually doesn't," I said.

The way the blood spread reminded me of a lotus flower. I imagined a room where my blood is photographed and framed.

I imagined drinking red wine, as though it was a gallery opening. This image made me feel safe, warm, the opposite of how my period so often felt to me.

The bright yet dull lights in the school cafeteria. How I loathed being there. The smell of chocolate milk and Styrofoam. Tomato soup. One of my school cafeteria memories really perplexes me. A sweatshirt was tied around the waist of khakis. The sweatshirt was navy. Navy blue was so popular then, too. (And do *not* wear navy blue with black unless you want the cool girls to make fun of you all day!) The girl wearing the sweatshirt walked out of the cafeteria while a group of kids laughed at her because of blood on her butt. Someone yelled, "You have blood on your butt!"

In the television show *PEN15*, in an episode called "Sleepover," the character Maya bleeds through her corduroys at a sleepover with four girls. Instead of telling them, she goes into the bathroom and rolls up a bunch of toilet paper to put in her pants. Throughout the night she continues doing this, until eventually the toilet clogs. One of the other girls finds it, starts pulling Maya's shorts down to see if she has her period. The mean girl notices a drip of blood on Maya's foot. The girls see the bloody toilet paper on the floor and freeze. Then, they begin throwing it at each other screaming, "Ew!"

"It's my blood!" Maya finally exclaims, putting the toilet paper back into her shorts. Instead of comforting Maya, the girls all run to her best friend, Anna, hugging her, saying they can't believe Maya hadn't told her she had her period, what a terrible friend Maya is, god forbid she wanted privacy.

In the next scene we see Maya in panicked tears, using the phone and asking to be picked up.

Watching this scene was like watching a horror movie. I remembered my cruelty toward others and their cruelty toward me at that age, the tension and manipulation and suffering through it, contributing to it. I remembered those calls to my mom—"Oh okay, I can't sleep over?"—pretending she was saying something on the other line that she wasn't saying. None of us had the emotional intelligence to work through our feelings of insecurity, inferiority.

We all shamed each other for having our periods, when having our periods was the most natural and healthy thing in the world. (Though if you'd told me that more than twenty years later, I'd be asking my boyfriend to look at my blood clots, I wouldn't have believed you.)

It's strange how periods were simultaneously coveted and made fun of. We wanted to get our periods to fit in, but we also used them against each other.

From Samantha Mann's essay "Seriously, I'm Kidding": "Another time we soaked a box of tampons in water dyed with red food coloring. We then took turns using the blow dryer to dry them out, which took quite a bit of time due to quality absorption. Once they dried we snuck out and hung them in a tree in the yard of this girl we hated."

Is my blood-on-your-butt fuzzy memory something I saw passively, or was I part of the incident? Was I the girl who tied the sweatshirt around her waist, or was I the girl who laughed at her? I will never know. It's more of a feeling, the memory. We are all every girl in high school. The girl who shames, the girl who gets shamed, and the girl who watches from the bleachers.

✦

"Your story won't work unless it's empathetic," I heard a guy with a beard tell another guy with a beard, at a coffee shop last week.

THE LINEN CLOSET

1932, Paris, France

My grandmother Simonne Lanowitz was born in 1920 in Paris and lived there until she was twenty-five. It always sounds so glamorous to me, but if she got her period when she was twelve, she may have had to wear sanitary bloomers, and no matter which way I turn the kaleidoscope, I just can't make that into glamour. The advertisement for the sanitary bloomers reads MADE OF ALL RUBBER, SELF-ADJUSTING, NO STRING, BUTTONS, OR PINS NEEDED. In all caps it reads A BIG SELLER! EVERY WOMAN WILL WANT ONE! The price was $13.50 for a dozen.

After World War II, in June 1946 when she was twenty-five, Simonne immigrated to New York City. She passed away in 2020, at age ninety-nine. Though we used to ask her many questions about her coming-of-age, I never asked her about her first period. I'm not sure she would have told me had I asked.

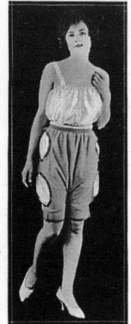
1961, Arlington, Massachusetts

Eileen was eleven. Their dad died the same year. "My mother
was businesslike. I passed out. It was extremely dramatic, clotty,
it was like something violent and horrible had happened to me.

My brother yelled, 'Mom,' and then she was 'oh you'll be okay,' almost smirky. I stayed home from school. I used an elastic belt and pad. I found the look really gross. I wouldn't have articulated it like a G-string but it looked obscene and in retrospect fucked with my sense of gender and how I felt about my body and how I looked. I never heard about PMS for about twenty years. I took drugs. Later. I took amphetamines when I felt the low blood sugar. Earlier I ate candy and got chubby. It would be complicated since I rejected having a female body, at least in the way in which it related to childbirth. I would have wanted a cultural conversation in which we talked about how it could be comfortable, how other people felt about it, what people meant when they said 'cramps,' which I never understood, and a conversation about gender. My alienation from having a body that enabled pregnancy but also had such powerful pleasure in its cycles deserved support and data and even humor that wasn't self-hating."

1964, Woodbridge, Connecticut

My godmother was thirteen. John F. Kennedy had been shot the year before, and Lyndon Johnson was sworn in. "I Want to Hold Your Hand" was all over the radio. Her period came later for her than her peers. She was given a menstrual belt with very little instruction on how to use it. She was never told anything about PMS and learned about it through a film shown (only to the girls) in sixth grade, but not boys. Her mother seemed embarrassed when asking her if she had any questions.

My godmother assumed her father never knew she got her period. She grew up to be a physician's assistant.

1965, Peekskill, New York

My aunt Maureen, the oldest of her four sisters, was fifteen, almost sixteen. She said her mother, my nana, took her into a dark, narrow hallway to a linen closet. She was told, "When you get your period, use this," and instructed to mark it on the calendar. She did so by drawing a circle so no one would know what it meant. She actually didn't know what it meant, either.

"It was actually freshman year in college that I learned from roommates that you could be pregnant if you don't get your period. This was at a time when my period was late, and I was sure I was pregnant . . . but I hadn't even had sex . . . a roommate explained it all to me.

"So college was when I put it all together but not until I wanted to get pregnant did I realize or think about how my body worked."

She vowed not to make her daughter, my cousin, feel shame and secrecy around her period.

My mom bought my cousin a teapot when she got her period.

"A teapot?" I texted. "That's so random."

"Yeah, congratulations, you're a woman now—here's a teapot!" my cousin said.

"It was cute!" my mom argued.

Apparently, I was at Pier 1 with my mom when she chose this teapot. It had a picture of a cat on it.

1967, Lake Geneva, Wisconsin

My mother-in-law was thirteen. She remembers escalating civil unrest associated with the Vietnam War. Young people were listening to the Beatles and the Rolling Stones, floating around on LSD. Hippies were having peace protests and wearing flower power pins.

"My own mother, who went to school in a one-room schoolhouse, had thought she was dying and was scared to tell her mother. I do have a memory of severe cramps my first few periods and feeling really wiped out. My mother basically told me *suck it up because you are going to have to deal with this for a long time.*

"So that's what I did . . . sucked it up and carried on."

My mother-in-law's last period was on her fiftieth birthday. She said that what she knows now that she didn't know then is that menopause is very freeing. She doesn't think anymore about her monthly cycle and that in itself is a relief.

1969, Peekskill, New York

My mom lived with her four sisters and three brothers, and she was the third oldest. She remembers President Nixon and how she loved the Beatles song "Michelle" so much that she pretended it was written for her.

For her first period, she used a menstrual belt. Her mother didn't show her how; her older sister, Maureen, did. She used the belt until sometime around 1973 when adhesive pads came on the market. She too remembers that my nana kept the pads and belts in the linen closet.

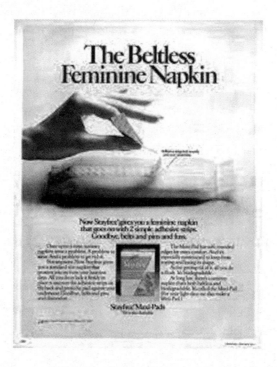

"My periods had such pain I didn't tell anyone about. I would cry in bed holding my stomach, trying not to let anyone know, even your dad. I thought it was normal 'cause no one talked about it. When I had your brother, I realized my early labor was exactly like my menstrual pain. I couldn't believe it. I missed many activities and times with friends due to canceling because of the pain. I wish I had talked to my mom but I'm not sure she knew what to do, either."

When I asked my mom if she ever took Advil or other pain medication for the pain, she responded: "No one ever advised ibuprofen and only much later in my life did I realize how much it helped."

I sent my mom a screenshot of a pencil drawing of the belt connected to a pad, labeled THE HOOSIER SANITARY BELT, asking, *like this?*

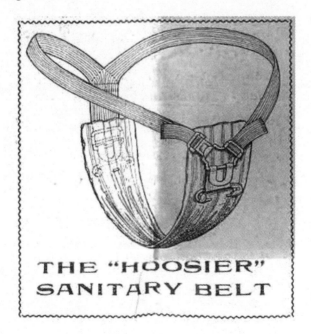

THE "HOOSIER" SANITARY BELT

She wrote back, "Ugh, I guess so."

"Why 'ugh'? Bad memories?"

"Yes. Probably wore the same belt for years. You had to make sure it was not sticking out of your pants . . . it was like having two pairs of underwear on. Felt like a diaper. Always worried boys could tell."

1976, Peekskill, New York

My aunt Bernadette was seventeen. She said: "Your nana's favorite line when I asked her to talk to me about menstruation or sex (the 'birds and the bees' as we called it) was: *You have time.* I remember so well hiding a tampon in my sleeve constantly when going to the bathroom, at school, or at rehearsal, etc., from sixteen and throughout my adult life. Mainly, though, I felt vulnerable.

"It took me a long time to realize how devastating one's period could be psychologically/mentally. I was never affected by my period physically besides being bloated, but emotionally I was a mess. Crying jags. Major despair. Oversensitive, etc. It was only when I was an adult and talking with my friends, or sisters, when we compared notes about our periods—usually when we started weeping about something!—that I discovered other people suffered psychologically/mentally as much as I did."

1977, San Diego, California

Rhonda was almost sixteen years old. "My mother had threatened to take me to the doctor because I hadn't started yet and she worried something was wrong with me. Luckily, I began in time because the thought of going to a gynecologist was unthinkable to me at that point. Jimmy Carter. *Roots* on TV. Elvis died. *Saturday Night Fever.* Fleetwood Mac *Rumours* over and over. Peter Frampton. I had rage and tears each month. Boyfriends knew to be sensitive at those times."

1977, West Linn, Oregon

Zach was eleven. "Disco was happening and I remember really being into KISS, because I was fascinated by guys wearing makeup and screaming. My dad was not around. My mom made a big deal out of it . . . a special lunch. She kept referring to my sister and me as 'women,' which felt odd because I was just eleven. She also got us douche kits when we were nine and ten, so I guess she was in a hurry for us to grow up. As a kid there were no symptoms that I remember. When I was older, if I started being obsessed with cleaning the house, crying, and feeling horny, I knew it was PMS. No matter what anyone says, I would never look back on my period as some transition into anything great. I wish I'd known that it was okay to think of my period as a monster instead of feeling like I had to embrace it as something wonderful."

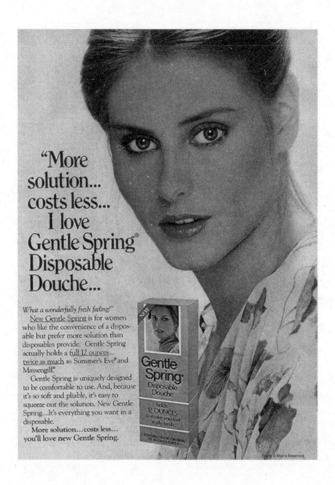

1983, Albany, New York

Sari was eighteen and a college freshman. It was the same year she heard "Holiday" by Madonna for the first time. Also, the Talking Heads' "Burning Down the House." It was the Reagan years.

"It was a doozy and lasted like twenty-two days. I had gotten a diaphragm (!) from Planned Parenthood at sixteen. That's right: I knew how to insert a diaphragm before I ever had occasion to use a tampon. A few months later I would undergo a laparoscopy that would reveal I had severe endometriosis and polycystic ovary syndrome. I wish I'd known that you don't have to suffer like I did. Hell, I wish someone would have just listened to me. I was dismissed again and again. Two different male doctors told me that what I experienced was just what it was to be a woman—that because I got my period late, I just wasn't used to it. I did not learn about PMS from doctors. I learned about it from friends. I suffered terrible PMS, usually for about half of each cycle, until I had a partial hysterectomy at forty-three."

1985, Mountlake Terrace, Washington

Erika was almost twelve. "OMG it was an amazing year for movies for someone my age. *Desperately Seeking Susan* with Madonna was out and I saw it in the theatre like five times with my BFF. *Pee-wee's Big Adventure* came out that year. *The Color Purple. Just One of the Guys* came out that year, a movie about a girl dressing up like a guy and I was obsessed with the girl in it and was starting to understand why. I loved *Teen Wolf* too because Michael J. Fox was the shit. For some reason, there were a lot of movies about transformation. I remember sending a tape to my friend Katy singing 'Crazy for You' by Madonna. We were a little gay for each other. I also remember Stevie Wonder and Dionne Warwick's 'That What Friends Are For' during choir at school.

"My mom was such a weirdo about it and it was kind of traumatizing. I called her at work and she didn't have anything for me at the house and acted very inconvenienced by my call. It was very emotional and I cried on the phone and I remember she seemed really annoyed. What bothered me the most at the time was that she didn't seem to understand why I felt lost and alone, and pretty rejected actually. She had a hard time putting herself in someone else's shoes and still does to this day. I hung up and called my mom's best friend, who helped me out with a pad and was really sweet about it. She made it seem like it was a rite of passage and was very comforting. I'm glad she was there for me, and it really helped me see how limited my mom was in dealing with independence or separation of any kind! My mom's friend took me to Arby's to celebrate, which was kind of cool. I had a French dip and a root beer.

"I told my brother and he sang the birthday song but 'Happy period to you!' At the end he said, 'And many more,' and my dad said something like, 'You don't know how right you are about that!'"

1988, Pittsburgh, Pennsylvania

Jamie got her first period a few months before her thirteenth birthday and remembers listening to the Smiths, Suzanne Vega, the Cure, and Billy Bragg.

"When I was in college I was out to lunch with my mom and my aunt and I was complaining about being *really* irritable (I probably said 'bitchy') during the lead-up to my period, which is when they told me my maternal great-grandmother had died by suicide postpartum and my grandmother (their mom) had attempted suicide postpartum and that there may be a connection between postpartum issues and PMS/PMDD (which wasn't a thing any of us named back then). This was the first I was hearing of any of this and I was *so pissed* at them for keeping it from me for so long. I had been menstruating for six years by then and felt like that knowledge really would have helped earlier. I've since been prescribed Lexapro, which has helped *so, so* much."

1992, Glens Falls, New York

My cousin Megan (the one who was gifted the cat teapot from my mom) got her period when she was ten, almost eleven, at our uncle's wedding. We were both wearing poofy dresses with huge floral prints on them. Her older brother noticed it first. He became a doctor, so maybe he was more attuned, even then. He told their mom.

"I developed much earlier than the majority of my friends and was the first to get my period by a few years. This resulted in my having a lot of shame around my body, my sexuality, and my menstruation. Growing up I used to always be so worried that I was going to bleed through my pants, show that I had my period, or even show my tampon string—especially when in a bathing suit. So I was constantly checking and sometimes I feel like those worries just consumed my thoughts. Those thoughts can take away from the carefree childhood everyone should have, right?!"

1994, Pittsburgh, Pennsylvania

Asmeret was fourteen. "All I remember is that I had just come home from a summer of traveling the country for dance competitions and was crushing on a dancer boy whom I was waiting to get a letter from. Still waiting for the letter. My mother was at work when I got my period, so I called her. In an effort to avoid her nosy coworkers, I remember her discreetly trying to explain to me where the hygienic products were located. I never told my father. Everything I learned about PMS I learned from my eighth grade life sciences teacher and by watching the movie *My Girl*. I wish someone had told me that your own saliva removes bloodstains. That would have saved me a lot of pairs of underwear."

1995, Klamath Falls, Oregon

Kristen was thirteen. "It was a big year for me personally because I started wearing contacts and went vegetarian. Two years prior, we'd had a random doublet earthquake in Klamath Falls (magnitudes 5.9 and 6.0) and ever since then, anything seemed possible. In April, 168 people were killed and hundreds injured in a domestic terrorist truck bombing in Oklahoma City.

"If supplies were low, I did not ask my mom to get more. Too embarrassing! Instead, I *made my own period products* using layers of toilet paper and Scotch tape which, in hindsight, is approximately ten thousand times more embarrassing than just asking someone for a tampon. Also, my homemade solutions didn't work very well, and I bled through them and it was a mess."

1996, San Diego, California
Vanessa was twelve. "The Spice Girls were a thing, and the O. J. Simpson trial was over but everyone was obsessed with making O.J. references. My dad wasn't around. My mom and aunt and sister were at my house. I remember it was the evening, and I came out of the bathroom low-key excited to announce that I had just gotten my period. I was pretty ecstatic about it, actually. I hated being a kid. I wanted to be a grown-up so bad, and the fact that I had gotten my period was proof that I wasn't a kid anymore. I think my mom and aunt were pretty chill about it and made sure I knew what to do. They made me some tea and gave me Motrin. I think I remember my mom turning to my aunt and saying, 'It's about to get worse.' I was already so insufferable. One day (within a year of getting my

first period) I decided to try out a tampon. I couldn't make sense of the instruction manual and I was being rushed out of the house because I was late to church, so I just inserted the entire thing inside me (with the cardboard applicator still attached) and hoped I got it right. Turns out sitting on a hardwood church pew for an hour with a cardboard applicator inside you is excruciating."

1998, Burlingham, New York

Jessica was growing up in Roslyn, New York, but was away at sleepaway camp.

"I don't think anyone ever talked to me about PMS, but I had an idea from pop culture. (*Clueless*, for example, stands out in my memory.) I think the main thing I wish I knew was that I could pay attention to my body to understand when I was getting my period, or that I could track days and get an idea of when I would get it. Obviously cycle-tracking apps didn't exist back then, but I think it was like always a surprise when I got my period for several years. I also think all the language around getting your period in the magazines I read was either embarrassing stories (getting your period in white pants at school or whatever) or super technical and how to deal with it. It was always presented as a total inconvenience and annoyance, which like it is, but I wonder how much the cultural narrative around periods shaped how I felt about it.

"Also, there was a huge stigma in my friend group around

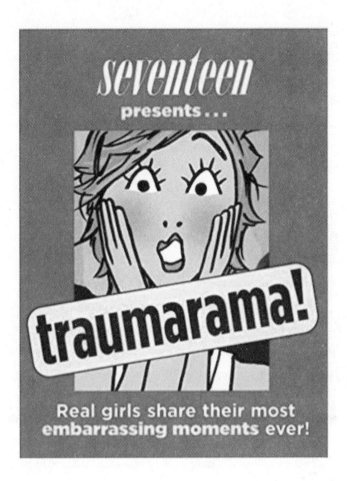

tampons. Like it was a *huge* deal to use them. I remember my friend's mom could not believe that I could figure out how to put a tampon in on my own. I never even told my mom I started using them. I just took them from her bathroom. But I definitely remember at the time being kind of surprised that

my friends didn't understand their bodies enough to instinc-
tively know how to use a tampon and the way they were all
acting about it made me scared and gave me this weird sense
of taboo. These are the same friends that now think menstrual
cups and even tampons without applicators are insane sooo I
guess maybe that says something about the culture where I'm
from."

2000, California

Cortney remembers the new millennium, the Bush vs. Gore
recount, mad cow disease, the dot-com bubble burst, and the
temporary retirement of her passion for Blink-182.

"I only remember not getting my first period. I had been
expecting my period every day since the age of ten after learning about it in school. When I was fourteen, my mom said, 'If
you don't get your period by the time you're fifteen, we'll go
to the doctor.' I secretly hoped it wouldn't come, that I would
go to the doctor and find out that I'd never have to get it. But
I did. Just before the 'deadline' and I don't remember a thing.
The first time I used a tampon was in a gas station bathroom
while on a family road trip. It was an emergency so my mom
handed me one of her O.B. tampons without the applicator.
She didn't explain how to insert it so I just closed my eyes
and tried to shove it in without touching anything. It hurt so
I freaked out and threw it away and stuffed my undies with a
wad of toilet paper.

"PMS was mentioned in health class a few times, but briefly and without detail. PMS became an abstract concept that boys abused to bully girls. I wasn't able to recognize or identify any PMS symptoms until I was an adult and had gone through enough periods to be my own personal expert. A couple years after I started my period, I went through a lot of instability and was no longer living at home. The inner turmoil I experienced then was mixed in with PMS symptoms and it all felt the same. I thought it was who I was. At eighteen, I started struggling with acne. I went to a doctor who prescribed birth control as medicine after he said, 'It doesn't look that bad' without even looking at my skin up close. The pills did nothing except make me gain twenty pounds and feel crazy because the extra hormones were combining with the mood swing side effect caused by my steroid asthma inhaler. I was unhinged, lashing out at friends, and had no one to turn to. After reading the side effects listed on my prescriptions more closely, I quit both, stabilized into a 'normal' cycle of PMS, and suffered on with my acne. I wish I'd known PMS can happen before and during and after your period, leaving you like one week a month of feeling all right. Symptoms can be different every time and may seem unrelated at first. They feel like unexplained microexperiences, like difficulty concentrating or losing coordination or forgetfulness, which are hard to even notice until the debt builds up and crushes you."

2000, *Bowling Green, Kentucky*

Stephanie was eleven. "I remember dancing to 'Thong Song' by Sisqó at my twelfth birthday party wearing a pad, feeling like a baby and a woman all at once. That was the year of the hanging chad debacle and the first year I started becoming aware of politics: my family was a blue bubble in a red state. I remember Napster blowing up, JLo's Grammys dress, and Britney's VMAs performance with that sparkly nude bodysuit. I was surprised because it felt like this mythical, huge moment I couldn't imagine happening to me. I told my mom and she hugged me. Later that night there was a bouquet of flowers in my room from her. A couple months later, in a golf cart on a golf course, just me and my dad, my dad said, 'I heard you became a woman,' and I told him to never talk to me about it ever again. He apologized and I remember bitching out my mom about telling him. Looking back, I can see his face so clearly and how torn he was about how to approach it or not and how he realized he'd made a mistake bringing it up. It's funny but it also makes me sad.

"No one had ever talked to me about PMS. I don't remember PMS symptoms until I was in high school and they were pretty intense. I didn't do anything about it except write in my journal and have panic attacks in my room. I recently found my high school journal and there are literal tear stains still on the paper on the pages where I wrote about how out of control

I felt during one of those times. I have no idea where I learned the term but at one point I wrote, 'Maybe it's PMDD or maybe I'm just insane.' I wish someone would have explained the menstrual cycle in a clear, direct way: the ovulatory phase, the luteal phase, etc., and what is happening during each. I wish someone would have told me that hormones control everything and a period is not some secondary random thing that people with uteruses just have. You literally have a different body every week. I could have understood myself so much better so much sooner."

2001, *Mountain View, California*

Audrey was in sixth grade, age twelve. "I don't remember my mom's reaction exactly, but shortly afterward she gave me a little clay figurine of a woman—painted in pastels, maybe with a butterfly?—with the date written in Sharpie on the bottom. I don't remember when I learned about PMS at all, actually. Most likely a joke was made in a sitcom and my mom explained it to me then. I do remember in first grade or so being told by a classmate that his sister told him women bleed out of their vaginas and I was positive he was lying.

"I use a menstrual cup now, which I first read about in Inga Muscio's *Cunt: A Declaration of Independence*—actually I think I read it the same year I performed in *The Vagina Monologues.*

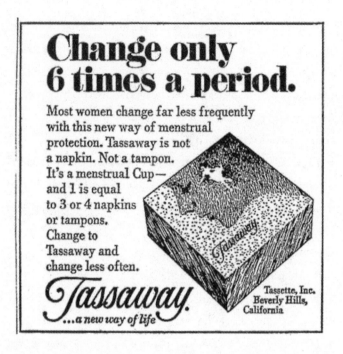

"Muscio encourages you to become familiar with your own menstrual blood (all your secretions, really), and I wish someone had told me as a preteen that menstrual blood is not something to be freaked out by, that it's pretty cool to shed remnants of what could have held a baby, but then again, I don't know if I would have listened then. Like what I *really* wish had happened was that someone had explained to me that the white cis hetero patriarchy is scared of women and their period blood and that's why periods feel inherently shameful, why they pour blue liquid instead of red in all the pad and tampon commercials, etc. But I didn't have anyone

in my life at that time who questioned the world order like
that."

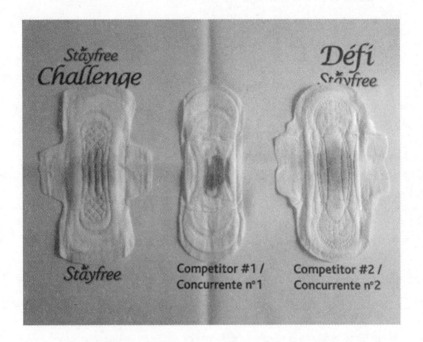

2002, Plymouth, Minnesota
Claire was fourteen. "I listened to ska and punk at my older
brother's urging (The Ramones, Bad Religion, Reel Big Fish,
Less Than Jake, Squirrel Nut Zippers, AFI, Black Flag, etc.),
and was doing my best to make being Lutheran cool by buying
Point of Grace and Five Iron Frenzy CDs. I was shocked that
no one told me it would/could look brown rather than red, but
it was just the first of so many things no one told me. I had

learned from a friend's unexpected period at my home the previous summer that 1) we have two holes, and 2) that a tampon
shouldn't feel like 'a giant wedgie.' My learning to use a tampon
was admittedly a bit slow but more successful than her unin-
tended butt plug experience."

2002, Chatham, New York
Noelle went to my high school but was a couple years younger
than I was. She used wadded-up toilet paper (many of us did!)
for the first year of her period, when she was fourteen.

"Destiny's Child was blowing up the music scene, and I was
all about it. There was a store called Weathervane at the Cross-
gates Mall that everyone shopped at. I had two or three shirts
from there that I wore on the regular. I got it at home and
remember trying to tell my body that I wasn't ready yet and
maybe it was just a mistake that it was happening already. But
it was the real deal. I didn't tell my mom for over a year. I felt
ashamed of my body and turning the corner into womanhood,
so I hid it. No one talked to me about PMS or my period. The
only information I had was from a video in fourth grade and
a pamphlet they gave us with some random info on it. I didn't
notice any PMS symptoms until I was more of an adult. I never
had cramps or felt overemotional until my midtwenties. Both
got progressively worse. I wish I'd known that your hormones
fluctuate and it's okay to stay home from social events to take
care of yourself. And that you shouldn't be ashamed of your

body's natural functions and feel the need to hide them. I spent so much time and energy keeping my period a secret from my family and I don't even know why. I was scared to admit I was human, I guess?"

2002, Cincinnati, Ohio
Sarah was twelve.

"I don't remember my parents having any reaction at all. I was raised Catholic—private Catholic K–8 program into Catholic all-girls high schools—which means I learned early on to associate my body with shame. I abjected myself, didn't want to talk about my body or its functions, especially not with my parents. I was too ashamed even to ask my older sister about it, and she's my best friend!

"I wish someone had told me I didn't have to suffer so much! It took many years of Google searches and talking to people to learn that I bleed more than the average menstruating person, cramp worse, and suffer a serious spike in depression right before my period, and that these are treatable symptoms. I had no idea that things like my coordination difficulties, forgetfulness, and self-image paranoia can be related to premenstruation. I spent so much time feeling like a wimp for not suffering with more grace, like it seemed everyone else was, but it turns out we were experiencing different things—and none of us should accept unbearable pain as simply part of the womb-haver's experience anyway. That's some Eve/original sin bullshit."

2003, Marlboro, New Jersey
Courtney had just turned fourteen.

"It felt like we were still very much embroiled in the fallout from 9/11—there was still a lot of anxiety around terrorism, including personal fear because my father worked downtown. High school was just about to start and I remember still tensing up in class freshman year when I would hear low or loud airplanes fly by. The Iraq War had started earlier that year and dominated the news cycle. I had a habit of checking Snopes.com when I'd get home from school to see what people were posting under a category called Rumors of War. In terms of pop culture, I remember going to see *Freaky Friday* and *Pirates of the Caribbean* in the theater that summer, running around the boardwalk at Point Pleasant while '21 Questions' by 50 Cent played on the sound system, and being absolutely feverish over the prospect of the Yankees entering the postseason. I also have a vivid memory of finding out John Ritter died one of the first few days of school while I was in history class.

"I told my mother immediately—rather, I screamed for her from the downstairs bathroom. I was crying and already running late to meet a friend at the Freehold mall for some unsupervised back-to-school shopping. I don't remember her precise reaction beyond telling me it was okay and trying to get me to calm down. I was crying but not entirely sure why I was crying. I asked her to bring me a tampon, but she refused and said I needed to start with pads. I don't remember telling my dad but I do remember his telling me I was lucky to have been educated and known what to expect (they bought me that American Girl book, *The Care and Keeping of You*, when I was in fourth grade—it was a long five-year wait between the education and the experience), and told me a story about how his mother's mother apparently did not tell her. She just saw blood in the toilet one afternoon while playing at her best friend's house and fainted. Her friend's mother had to explain the entire thing to her.

"I used a pad at my mother's behest. I was mortified because I'd borne witness to my best friend getting bullied on the bus in seventh grade when her pads fell out of the front zipper pocket of her backpack. The prospect of having those cumbersome pads accompany me every day at high school brought me a lot of shame. I was warned (by whom, it's unclear) that keeping pads in your purse was a no-go and I'd be better off hiding them in my shoes. I hid them in my shoes until the day the boys on the bus tore my shoes off and threw them down the aisle, pads falling to the ground like leaves. I finally started using tampons after I started having sex at sixteen.

"I was told about PMS but in such gentle, lamblike terms. I assume that was done so as not to frighten me? I remember being told—maybe by the school nurse or the health teacher or the American Girl book—that there would be irritability and cramps but in such a way that it was made to seem like a bubble bath and a square of chocolate could fix what ailed me. That was obviously bullshit. Also I hate bubble baths.

"I treated the physical symptoms of PMS with ibuprofen and a hot-water bottle. But I did nothing to acknowledge or treat the emotional and psychological symptoms of PMS. All my symptoms got far less severe when I went on birth control at sixteen, but when I had to come off it at twenty-five and started getting serious symptoms again, I felt like I was behind on developing proper coping mechanisms.

"I feel like I have better coping and treatment mechanisms now that would have been really useful then, both for pain management and emotional relief. (If only I could hand a Post-it note with the words "masturbation + CBD" written on it across time to younger me. Sigh.) I wish I knew then that it actually wasn't a big deal and that it makes little sense to hold myself up to arbitrary yardsticks, like the ages of relatives or Judy Blume protagonists."

2003, *Chino Hills, California*

Lisa got her period a few weeks after her twelfth birthday.

"In politics the war on Iraq began, which was mega in the States. My taste in music had gone from Avril Lavigne, Good Charlotte, Simple Plan to freak dancing music like 'My milkshake brings all the boys to the yard' to 'I like the way you do that right thurrrr (right thurrr)' and 'I got the magic stick, I know if I can hit once, I can hit twice.' I don't think these lyrics are appropriate for any twelve-year-old child to listen to today but these were the hottest tunes playing on the radio 24/7 back then and I couldn't get these lyrics out of my head even if I wanted to.

"I remember sitting on the toilet when I noticed a tinge of blood on my underwear. It took a minute to register that I had started my period and I wadded up a piece of toilet paper and placed it on top of my underwear. I scurried over to my diary and wrote these exact words, '*OMG I started my period!!*' Then I waited for my mom to come home from work and broke the news to her. She was more excited than I was and rushed me to the grocery store to stock up on the essential period pack: pads, tampons, and chocolate.

"Nobody ever talked to me about PMS. I learned about periods, sex, and PMS from a book I picked up at a local bookstore when I was probably eleven or twelve years old. I can't remember the title of the book but I used to hide the book in my underwear drawer or underneath my dresser and read it to myself in secret when nobody was home. It felt shamefully wrong for me to know about sex, relationships, and 'adult' things in my household. Maybe it was a part of my Korean culture that we never talked about sex or mental health but there is an underlying shame and guilt pertaining to the topic.

"The first PMS symptom I ever got was absolutely brutal. I remember feeling sick with the flu. I had body aches, chills, a high fever, and these god-awful pains in my stomach that I now know as period cramps. I was crawling on all fours to my bathroom because I thought I was going to puke from the nausea. After sitting on the toilet I discovered my first real 'heavy' period. This period came a couple weeks after my initial 'spotting' incident and I had never seen so much blood inside the toilet bowl. I slapped the thickest pad I had onto my underwear and crawled back to my bed on all fours and slept the period pains away.

"The one thing I wish someone would have told me when I was young was the immense impact that my period would have on my general well-being. That my PMS/PMDD symptoms can sometimes become so severe that it'll affect my mood, my thought process, my behavior, my mental health, and my energy levels so much to the point that I become a different person. I also wish someone would've told me that I should be diligent about monitoring my menstrual cycle like my life depends on it because it will have a negative impact on my relationships, work, and mental health. Forgetting that my period is coming around the corner is like forgetting to remember that the monthly fluctuations of the hormones inside my body can be the main cause for my irrationality, anxiety, depression, monstrous appetite, and self-loathing is because I am a woman and not put the blame on the rest of the world. (Even though I secretly do every. single. time.)"

2005, Vancouver, British Columbia

Mona was living in Vancouver after immigrating from São Paulo, Brazil. "It was one month before I turned seventeen. *Everyone*, including my younger sister, had already gotten their periods. I was sure it would never happen for me, and I saw a documentary on intersex people and was convinced I was one. Because I waited so long for it, I remember exactly what I wore, and when I saw it. I was in the bathroom of my new high school, having been taken out of the private school that I attended my whole life because of financial problems my dad had, and I was wearing light-wash jeans. I told my mom and was entirely shocked that it was more a river of blood than the couple of droplets I had yearned for for so long. I used pads. Brazilians *never* use tampons."

2005, Humble, Texas

Kellie got theirs the summer before eighth grade. "I have a vivid memory of getting it and being devastated. I had not yet come to terms with my gender variance, but absolutely hated all things 'girl.' To me, this was another horrifying step toward growing up and becoming feminine. I went to a private Christian school and lived a very sheltered existence. My parents were very overprotective and we didn't talk much, if at all, about personal topics like puberty, sexuality, etc. I wish I had known more about gender, and known that my feelings were valid and real. I wish I had known that there were other folx who, like me, felt like hitting puberty and beginning to become more feminine was not something they wanted. And more than anything, I wish that I had had the words to talk about what I was feeling and find the support I needed to navigate what these changes meant for my body and my future."

2005, Madison, Connecticut

Julia was thirteen and sixteen. "Like many people, I think I actually got my 'first period' twice. once when I had no idea what was happening, and the second time when I thought to myself: finally. The 'first time' I was in eighth grade (age thirteen) in Madison, Connecticut. It was 2005. The second time, I was in tenth grade (age sixteen), and still in Madison, but it was 2008. I was the last of my friends to get my period. I didn't get it again until I was in college, but I knew that I'd gotten it 'for real' that second time. The female body, man. The second time I got my first period I was obsessed with running and fell in love with my high school track coach (a woman! the horror).

"No one talked about PMS growing up. I have zero recollection of anyone discussing it growing up. I have horrible PMS now and have at many times thought I have PMDD. At fifteen, I had an ultrasound on my pelvic region to see if I had endometriosis or any cysts that needed to be addressed (this was largely because I still hadn't gotten my period again). I remember this moment vividly for a few reasons: the ultrasound wand had to penetrate me (I'd never had sex), and the woman who performed it was a classmate's mom. She was really uncomfortable and could tell I was crying, it was awful. Midol is amazing, exercise around the days just prior to your period is very difficult, and being gentle with both your physical and mental self during those days leading up to your period is essential."

2006, Orlando, Florida

Halle was living in Knoxville, Tennessee, but got her period in Orlando at a carnival at the themed Embassy Suites hotel. She was twelve.

"I remember the night before I started, I went swimming and I could not for the life of me stop swimming, I never wanted to get out of that water. I got my period early the next morning. My mom was amazing. I was mortified to tell her; I remember praying on the toilet to god to 'take it back.' I'd wanted a period so long and when I got it, I realized that my life really would change. I felt tied down. But my mom hugged me and took me to breakfast after we got everything cleaned up. Tampons or menstrual cups were strictly forbidden. Mostly because of toxic shock fears, but also for religious reasons. Virginity was an expected standard in my southern household, and any insertion seemed like a gateway to other sexual exploration.

"For about a year before, we read a book together called *The Period Book*, and we prepared for PMS and the mood swings that would come with it. My mom was always sympathetic about it and talked to me openly. We bonded over this a lot. She was a safe space. I remember vividly the fear I felt telling my dad or brother about it. I wish I knew how much my period would affect my mental health. We have a history of clinical depression and bipolar disorder in my family, and periods make all my triggers twenty times worse."

2006, Houston, Texas

Catherine was fourteen. "I just remember eating lunch alone in the library while listening to the *Rent* soundtrack (the *movie* not musical LMAO) also listening to *lots* of the *Wicked* soundtrack and singing it *so loud* as my mom drove me to my new school where I had no friends. I called my mom from school to tell her and when I got home there was a box of junior tampons in front of my bedroom door, and we never spoke of it again. I told her not to tell my dad because I was embarrassed. My friends showed me how to put a tampon in and told me I was 'too hairy' to see the hole, LOL. I used pads because I was too scared to insert a tampon until I had to go to my friend's beach house in Galveston and knew then I would need to suck it up and use a tampon so I could swim, which I did. I feel I'm too moody to ever tell what's what. Also, I have PCOS so I'm super irregular and rarely have a period. I wish I'd known it's not normal to miss your period for eight months even if you're a virgin . . . Go to the doctor, girl."

2019, Anacortes, Washington

My cousin Bella was seventeen.

"I remember that Billie Eilish came out with a new album that year, which I listened to nonstop. Donald Trump was still president. I was the only person I knew of my age that hadn't gotten it. When my friends talked about their periods, I never told anyone that I hadn't had mine—I felt embarrassed of myself. I actually lied a few times, and acted like I had already had it. Well, maybe not lied—on the few occasions that my friends had talked about their periods with one another, I would sometimes nod and smile and laugh, like I could relate to what they were saying. I didn't want anyone to know that mine was so late. My mom and I went to see a doctor to make sure that everything was okay with my hormones and my body after I turned seventeen and still hadn't gotten it. I had to get my blood drawn, which was *much* more traumatic for me than any period I've ever gotten. I remember that the doctor mentioned that there was a small possibility that maybe I just didn't have a uterus. That really scared me, and I think scared my mom, too. Suddenly, I was way more concerned that there was something actually wrong with me. Everything ended up being completely normal though and I got my first period a few months later.

"My mom was so happy for me, she hugged me when I told her and smiled so big. She seemed to be so proud of me. My mom and I told my dad later that day, and he was really happy, too. They were both so open about it and didn't make it embarrassing for me at all, even though I felt a little embarrassed myself.

"I learned about PMS in fifth grade. I took a class at the Seattle Children's Hospital with my mom, my best friend, and her mom that taught young girls about puberty, sex, periods; the instructor touched on PMS, too. Even though I didn't get my period until six years after I took that class, I still think that it helped to open up the conversation for me as a younger girl and make it seem like a normal, exciting thing rather than a horrific, life-altering one. It made me more aware of the changes that were happening in my body, and made me feel less shame and embarrassment around it than I think I would have had if I didn't go to the class.

"My period is so irregular that it can be really hard for me to tell if I'm actually experiencing sadness and sensitivity and breakouts because I'm about to get my period, or just because I'm eighteen and still a teenager and sometimes just feel those emotions and symptoms out of the blue anyway. But whatever the case, it's never so extreme that I don't know how to cope. I'll usually just write a couple of pages in my journal, explaining how my day was and why I'm so angry or sad or annoyed. That really helps to ground me, I find.

"Although I haven't had my period for very long, I am definitely more open to talking about it with my friends, mom, etc. than when I first got it. I wish I had known that it is something that is completely okay to talk normally about! I am lucky to have such open parents that don't make it a big deal or something embarrassing, but when I first got it, I was still reluctant to talk about it to them and also to my friends. Now my friends and I more openly talk about getting our periods/how it affects us/the struggles of having a period. My friend and I were actually just recently talking about how we think it's so annoying how we still feel like we have to sneakily take tampons out of our backpacks when we have our periods at school. Why isn't it okay to just walk down the hallway holding a tampon? It's almost like when you see another girl taking a tampon out of her backpack and slipping it up her sleeve at school, you feel like you caught her. As if she failed to convince the entire world that periods don't exist. It's weird! For the most part, though, I don't really feel like there's anything that I'd wished I had known. I think that periods are finally getting more normalized (why they were not always a normal thing to talk about, I don't know), which is encouraging to see."

✦

1985
One year before I was born, Courtney Cox was the first person to say "period" on television, in a Tampax commercial. She is in a locker room, in a purple T-shirt and a different shade of

purple leggings. Her hair is very close to being a mullet. Behind her, two women are doing ballet. Courtney Cox played my least favorite character on *Friends*, but I have more respect for her now.

1987

In *Just as Long as We're Together*, arguably the best Judy Blume book (aside from *Summer Sisters*, of course), the narrator Stephanie gets her period on her birthday and is met with support from her teacher, plus her friends.

1993

My dad heard a joke about two musicians who only had $1.75 between them. One of the musicians said, "I know what we should do, get a box of Tampax."

The other responded, "What the hell are we gonna do with a box of Tampax?"

The first musician said, "Don't you read the magazines? We can go horseback riding, we can go swimming, we can go ride bicycles and eat ice cream."

1996

There's a chapter in *The Vagina Monologues* by Eve Ensler called "I Asked a Six-Year-Old Girl."

If your vagina got dressed what would it wear?

Red high-tops and a Mets cap worn backwards.

1997

The light-purple sports bra was my first bra. I don't remember where we purchased it, or why I am saying "we"—only that I'm assuming my mother was with me. I remember wearing it around the house, excited. I was wearing it with shorts, probably Umbros. I went upstairs to my mom's room and she told me to put a shirt on before my dad and brother came home.

I don't remember why it was light purple. I don't think I liked purple, though, come to think of it, I had a purple blow-up chair in my bedroom. Metallic purple and green beads hanging in front of my bed. I tried on my best friend's older sister's purple dress to wear to the Queen of Hearts Dance. When I tried it on in front of everyone—my mom, my friend, her sister, their mom—I didn't know how to stand to have good posture. My mom said, "Are you sticking your breasts out?" And I didn't know if I was or not. So maybe I did like purple. That's the thing about memory: just because you want to have been the kind of teenager who didn't like purple doesn't mean you were.

1998

Age eleven, lying across the couch. Was I taking a nap? Hearing my mom on the phone telling someone, "She got her period but said she didn't." A sort of laughter. Actually, according to an old notebook I was twelve, but I wrote that entry in my twenties. I'm positive I was eleven. I had my period and my mom took me aside and told me to wrap my pads up better; otherwise they smelled. I felt embarrassed.

But there's a hole in the memory. I remember leaving blood-stains on this light-brown couch with a tiny navy blue pattern on it. But the couch I was lying on while she was on the phone was dark navy, midnight blue, and it wouldn't have been possible to leave those sort of bloodstains on it. It is possible I had my period on the beige couch a few weeks (days? months?) earlier, and this memory of hearing my mom on the phone was a completely different day and I am conflating the two couch memories. What season did I get my period? Why do I only remember the stain on the couch? Was there snow? Was it near my birthday? Was it a school day? Only the stain remains in my mind.

2006

In Williamsburg, Brooklyn, in my salad days, I heard the Dolly Parton song "PMS Blues" at a bar that no longer exists: *Most times I'm easygoing, some say I'm good as gold / But when I'm PMS I tell ya, I turn mean and cold.*

2009

My Little Red Book, edited by Rachel Kauder Nalebuff, an eighteen-year-old, was released from Hachette. Rachel had begun collecting "first period" stories when she got her period at thirteen. She told *The New Yorker*: "Sensing my embar-rassment, my great-aunt Nina told me a story that put it all in perspective. She had gotten her period just as she was about to be strip-searched on a train fleeing Nazi-occupied Poland. Incredibly, she hadn't told anyone about it until our conversation. I was taken aback. How could she keep such a dramatic story to herself? Did other women in my family have similarly powerful stories and I just didn't know?"

2013

Thinx period underwear was launched, though it was a few years later when I tried it, after the ads targeted me aggressively. Finally, I found the moxie and money to order one pair of the high-waisted ones. There is no way, I thought, that these can hold all my blood on my heaviest day. But they did. I ordered two more pairs. Tony calls them my Stinks. *Are you wearing your Stinks?* he'll say.

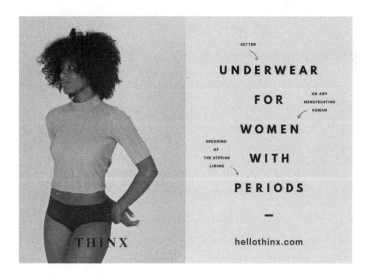

One night while doing laundry at my mom's, I showed them to her. She was in disbelief. "I would have *loved* these," she said, and I saw envy come over her the same way it had come over me when I learned about the period board game.

2014

Somehow I came across a Kickstarter for the Period Game. In their words: "The Period Game is a fun, positive, learning experience that teaches participants about what is happening within menstruating bodies and how to 'go with the flow.' It's pretty much impossible to play the game without saying words like 'period' and 'tampon,' making it a lot easier to talk about both in real life, and empowering the next generation to stop hiding tampons in their sleeves. Our mission is to make young people's first experience with menstruation a positive one, to help demolish the period stigma before it even starts." Obviously, I want to buy the game for Sadie. She loves board games, but maybe by buying this, I'm overcorrecting.

2015

A woman named Kiran Gandhi, also known by her stage name Madame Gandhi, ran a marathon in London, free bleeding. She didn't want to run with a pad chafing her thighs (and maybe falling out?) or a tampon plugged up her. "I decided to just take some Midol, hope I wouldn't cramp, bleed freely and just run. A marathon in itself is a centuries old symbolic act.

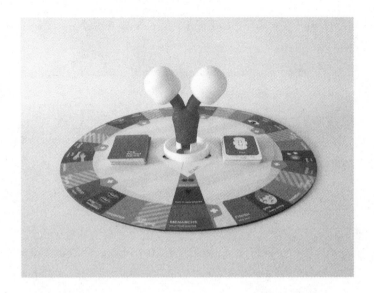

Why not use it as a means to draw light to my sisters who don't have access to tampons and, despite cramping and pain, hide it away like it doesn't exist?" she wrote in an article for Medium. "I was going through all these crazy thoughts and analyzing whether I was either a) a crazy chick who needs to just calm down and reach for an effing tampon or b) a liberated boss madame who loved her own body, was running an effing marathon and was not in the mood for being oppressed that day."

2016

The only person who has ever sent me a photo of their menstrual blood is a student from one of my classes who became a good friend. I'd been flying home from somewhere, and when the plane I was on landed and I turned on my phone, a text came through:

My period on the second day is literally a joke, captioning a photograph of red blood on the floor.

Did you just send me a picture of your menstrual blood?

Yah cause it fell in two perfect circles, that's never happened before.

2018

The documentary filmmaker Sindha Agha released a video essay on *The New York Times* titled "Birth Control Your Own Adventure," about her struggle with what ended up being endometriosis.

"I got my first period when I was eleven," she says, as an image of ketchup squirts onto a paper plate decorated with illustrations of colorful balloons. "My dad stayed home. He waved incense over my head and blasted Gregorian chants from the boombox. I was in so much pain." The subtitle to her video is *How my side effects made me four different people.* When she gets an IUD inserted on a doctor's recommendation, she describes the pain being so acute that she "hallucinates violent things happening to fruit."

Sindha quits her job and travels to Iceland, feeling called to visit a Nordic setting. But one day while driving, she feels nauseated, as if she is going to upchuck ice cream. "The sheep

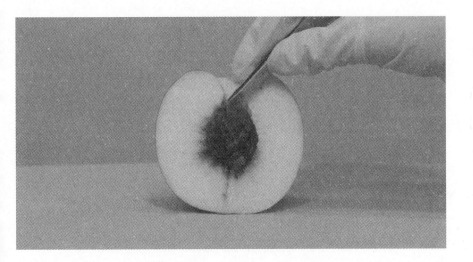

don't look well-meaning. The sky looks carnivorous. I don't feel real. I call my friend Stephanie. *Can you describe me to myself?*"

Back at the doctor, Sindha is told her IUD is causing PMDD. She's put on propranolol, something usually given to musicians, actors, and public speakers for its ability to treat anxiety symptoms activated by the sympathetic nervous system.

"Normal people probably don't medicate themselves to stay calm around Icelandic sheep," Sindha replies.

"I don't know what you mean by 'normal people,'" her doctor responds.

A pause. "Yes, you do."

Sindha has spent over a decade trying different hormonal contraceptives—and she's only twenty-four. Over email, she wrote me: "It all feels so unfair . . . PMDD, endometriosis, every other reproductive disorder women suffer from. Do you ever think, 'All this just so I can have a baby?!' Babies are great, but sometimes I find myself wishing there was some kind of opt-in they would've given me. Not sure I would have elected to have this reproductive system, with all its side effects and disorders. I've been considering going on an antidepressant part of the month for the PMDD window."

Her short film reached 12 million organic Facebook views, and has almost 900,000 views on YouTube. The film was later nominated for a Documentary Emmy.

2019

The essay "Notes on Bleeding and Other Crimes" was published in the collection *Notes to Self* by Emilie Pine. She opens with: "Famously, the trick to good writing is bleeding onto the page. I picture the male writer who coined this phrase, sitting at his typewriter, the blank sheet before him. What kind of blood did he imagine? Blood from a vein in his arm? Or a leg? Perhaps a head wound? Presumably it was not blood from a cervix. I have so much of this blood, this period blood, this pregnancy blood, this miscarriage blood, this not-pregnant-again blood, this perimenopausal blood. It just keeps coming and I just keep soaking it up."

2020

Sadie and I watched the new *Baby-Sitters Club* and Kristy, the tomboy, gets her period and Alicia Silverstone, who plays her mom, meets her with excitement, and her friends Claudia, Stacey, and Dawn give her a pad and wait for her outside the door. Kristy comes through the door and says she needs more cake. "Makes sense," the other girls say.

My mom and I were driving home from a restaurant and I mentioned the linen closet. She made a noise of negativity, as though she hated thinking about the linen closet.

"What's with you all and that linen closet?" I asked.

"Probably because our cat gave birth in there, and everything was bloody."

It's curious to me that neither my mom nor I can recollect any details of my first period. It's okay, though. My periods later more than made up for it.

THE NUGGET BETRAYAL

r/AskReddit: Ladies, what stupid thing did PMS make you cry about?

When Trader Joe's wine went from $2 to $3.

KFC was out of honey BBQ wings. I felt disrespected.

I touched my bird and he was fluffy and I cried because I felt so lucky to be able to pat it every day.

I cried for hours because I felt I wasn't a good enough mom to my cat for working long hours that day.

Went through the drive-thru at Chick-fil-A with my boyfriend at the time and ordered my usual chicken nugget meal with a sweet tea. On the way home, the motherfucker started to drink all of my sweet tea. I was looking forward to enjoying it with my chicken nuggets, so I burst into tears.

Cried on my birthday because my cheesecake slice wouldn't properly stand upright and then cried again because I cried over cheesecake.

Cried in the parking lot outside of my house when I opened my six-piece McNuggets box and only saw five. And by "cried," I mean I was full-on sobbing and mumbling incoherently about my nugget betrayal.

My boyfriend and I have been talking about adopting an older dog and I woke up early on a rainy morning to sit on our balcony and saw a guy walking his dog. From there, my brain went through "We can't have a dog, we have carpet everywhere, who's gonna clean up after it? They don't even like wearing those little shoes so it's too complicated when it rains and they get muddy paws!" Then I started crying because I was sad about not getting a dog and I crawled back into bed to tell him and instead of going through the logical explanation I'd just given myself, I bawled to my very sleepy boyfriend that "We can't have a dog, they don't wear shoes."

I couldn't get the wi-fi to work and it kept rejecting my password, so I grabbed a candy bar, curled up on an armchair, and cried myself to sleep in a ball while cuddling the candy bar.

I went to Tim Horton's to get a 10 pack of Timbits (doughnut holes) because I was really craving them. I asked for no plain ones because they're nasty. On my way home I opened the box and half were plain ones and I started crying and threw each plain one out the window as I drove home bawling.

My dog having the body shape of a kidney bean.

I was cranky and craving a cannoli so I complained to my fiancé about it. He stood up and said "ok" and started putting on his coat to go get me a cannoli. I cried because I was so happy to be getting a cannoli and because I felt so bad, I was making him do it. Was still crying when I ate the cannoli but damn it was good.

The worst of it had me sobbing at a pot of overcooked pasta and screaming at my husband about it being the worst thing that could have possibly happened while I proceeded to throw our entire dinner in the trash.

My wife started crying because the poached eggs on her eggs benedict were so soft and beautiful.

My cat doesn't know I love her.

We were out of peanut butter cups!!!

My boyfriend made me grilled cheese with garlic bread toast as the bread and I couldn't handle it. It tasted so good.

I wanted takeout and he brought home steamed dumplings instead of fried and I generally like steamed over fried but apparently had decided I wanted fried not steamed that day without telling anyone the details. Proper hysterics and dumplings were thrown up the stairs (yes *up* the stairs). It was dubbed the great dumpling incident of 2011.

I went to Jack in the Box to get 2 EGG and CHEESE CROISSANTS and then an extra 2 for my mom. Anyway, I was depressed and was starving after work, ordered my food and everything seemed to be in order . . . drove the 15 minutes home and opened my food. ALL FOUR SANDWICHES WERE SAUSAGE AND EGG ONLY BISCUITS. I started fucking screaming how I was 'fucking pissed off' and how much I 'hate my fucking life' and how I 'refuse to eat this shit' and 'everything always happens to ME' and proceeded to throw a sandwich on the counter. My mom just stared at me as I sobbed into the couch and she offered to drive and get me my egg and cheese croissants like I wanted . . . I just sobbed and said no, and I heated up a Lean Cuisine and cried myself to sleep. The next morning, I ate those fucking sausage and egg biscuits like nothing happened.

Christmas Eve a few years back. Came home after a long day and could hear that a lone goose was distantly honking in the night. I started crying because he was alone on Christmas.

My husband and I played Monopoly. I was winning and took almost all his money. I then realized he would starve to death if I took everything and I started bawling my eyes out. We had to stop playing. Next day we tried to continue but again the thought of my husband starving to death because he can't buy food made me cry my eyes out. Haven't played Monopoly ever since. That was ten years ago.

✦

In my twenties I might have fit into this Reddit thread. Now though, the group I lurk is not the one for "ladies" who cry from "PMS." The group where I have found my compatriots is called Werewolf Week and is another animal entirely—a vicious, aggressive, unfunny animal, an animal who destroys your garden.

PART TWO

AFTER WOMEN

The summer I began dating Tony, I received an email from GO *Magazine* wanting to list me as one of a hundred influential gay women. I'd read the email quickly, and at first thought it said GQ magazine, which made no sense.

I'm reaching out because you've been nominated among hundreds of prominent out lesbians for inclusion in our annual 100 Women We Love feature.

Was I prominent? Was I out? Was I a prominent out lesbian?

◆

When I was twenty-eight, I published an autobiographical novella about a relationship with a gay woman, exploring my queer identity, or whether I had one. I'd figured about fifty people would read the book, but it exceeded my expectations. It was 2014, Obama was president, and Instagramming books was relatively new. The dancing girl emoji was new. #TBR stacks were new. All of this contributed to the book thriving.

As the years went on, the book took on an identity and I floated above it, watching it happen. I'd get texts: "I'm listening to two women next to me uptown who are talking about *Women*." Readers would write to tell me that it helped them with their own identity and inspired them to come out, or that they wanted it back from their ex. It was photographed numerous times with pieces of jewelry, especially gold jewelry, and skin care products: oils, creams, toners. Authors speak of this all the time—that once the book is in the world, it doesn't belong to you anymore. Anne Lamott says of her cult fave *Bird by Bird* that to her it was a small little book; she'd written it in six months. I'd written mine in six months, as well.

An example of something that frequently occurred after I published *Women*: I'd meet a woman for drinks. The margaritas would get me lit. Halfway through our second round she worked into the conversation that she'd be paying. So we got more. She liked me okay, but when I was drunk enough to disclose I'd published a book called *Women*, her interest was obviously piqued. She wanted to know everything. What did the woman look like, how butch was she?

We walked toward the street we both lived on. She complimented my boots. We parted ways. She texted in the morning and I could feel she'd googled me. Now she was really interested. This turned me away. She invited me to drink wine with some old

wine-seller man. I declined. She invited me to Big Gay Ice Cream.
"As friends only!" she said, sensing my guardedness. Though she
lives on my street, I never bump into her, never see her again.

✦

Five years ago, I took the train ten hours to give a reading from
a new book in Montreal. It'd been two years since *Women* was
published, two years since I'd last read in Montreal. The room
was filled with queer women, queer haircuts, tote bags that
read MOTHER EARTH IS A LESBIAN.

"You have a very specific demographic," one of the book-
sellers said to me.

I had anticipated meeting someone that night, at least running into an acquaintance. A member of the audience. Maybe
they'd invite me to dinner or a drink or a party afterward. I
finished the reading and Q&A, waited a couple minutes,
browsing books, and left the bookstore alone. All the women
who'd watched me, who were so supportive of me and so attractive, were huddled in a group. They were friends; they were
a community.

It was bitter, epically cold. My phone wasn't set up for data
in Canada. I went to a Starbucks to get Wi-Fi, ate a choco-
late-covered graham cracker, a little drunk on the wine they'd
provided me before the reading. I looked at my Instagram,
a photo someone had posted of me reading, and I probably

posted a photo of myself. I walked back to my cousin's friend's place. I couldn't afford a hotel. It was freezing. Someone had told me everyone's apartment in Montreal is freezing. Somehow the cold made my loneliness more pronounced.

I slept in all my clothes: my tights and socks, a heavy sweater over a long-sleeved shirt. My grandmother had knitted me the sweater and by sleeping in it, I stretched it out and ruined it; when I woke up it had completely lost its shape.

✦

In September of 2017, I was invited to lunch with a renowned lesbian poet and they asked if I was dating a man or a woman. I wanted to say a woman, but I'd just left Tony's apartment where he was vacuuming his car. I'd been in the bathroom making sure I looked okay. He was excited about who I was going to lunch with. When I got back, we were picking his daughter up from school.

I stabbed my fork into my beet salad. (We were both eating beet salads. They paid for them because their publisher paid for them. It is the best salad in town; it comes with edible flowers and blue cheese crumbles.) I was wearing jeans and a T-shirt. A couple years earlier I would have dressed up, put on a dress or a shirt I perceived as sexy, but Tony, Sadie, and I had been at the park flying kites that morning, so I was in jeans and red T-shirt and black high-top Converse. They wore navy-and-white high-top Converse. I took a photograph of our sneakers.

"That's hilarious," they said, glancing at our shoes.

"Man," I answered.

One morning I see a cartoon in *The New Yorker* of two men looking at a tree. *Maybe it doesn't want to be identified*, one of the men says.

✦

In the past seven years or so, it seems like a lot of women around my age (okay, millennials, *there I said it*) have realized that maybe they were queer. It was especially popular if someone who was publicly "straight" went publicly "gay." Most of these women had married men in their twenties.

Going from queer icon to hetero is not nearly as fun as it looks to go from hetero to queer. Was I letting people down now that I posted photos of me, Tony, and Sadie in front of a Christmas tree? Flying a kite? Coloring Easter eggs?

"I can't believe you came out publicly as straight," one of my friends said when I posted the first photo of Tony and me to social media.

In an article for *The Guardian* titled "I'm queer no matter who I'm with. I won't define myself differently for your comfort," Ashley C. Ford writes: "Identifying as queer means being mistrusted, misunderstood, and, often, mislabeled for the rest of your life. Every time you date a new person, you have to come out again."

It reminds me of being in high school and a friend saying, "Do you play guitar?"

"No."

"You'd be cooler if you did," she said.

"I know."

"How does a person write truthfully about their life, when it isn't finished?" Molly Wizenberg asks in her memoir *The Fixed Stars*.

I've published four books; three before I was thirty, and it is impossible to write a book that represents you forever. Does anyone expect us to, though? Published books are sort of like marriage vows. You publicly state something, and later you change your mind, or you grow, or you divorce. Or the truth becomes more complicated.

✦

I wasn't sure how to respond to *GO Magazine*'s email. I figured the best thing to do was to be up front, so I wrote to the editor of the feature. *I don't identify as a lesbian and I'm in a hetero relationship but am 100% queer!* Except I had a typo, and instead of writing *100% queer*, I wrote *10% queer*.

Tony was out of town. I called him to tell him the news and about the typo, unsure of how he'd react about my being in the feature. I'd dated one other male four years back and his reactions to my writing and public persona were harsh and mean, making me a little gun-shy.

He laughed so hard.

The editor responded: *That doesn't affect anything! This features women who identify as lesbian or queer.*

They published my photograph in the magazine.

HORMONOLOGY

In my twenties I had a PC computer, and I remember how a bright red message often popped up on my screen: WARNING! YOU HAVE A VIRUS!!!!!!!

There were two options to click on: "Ignore and Continue" and something along the lines of "Deal with the Virus." Noelle, when she was my roommate, laughed over my shoulder every time I clicked on "Ignore and Continue." I treated my body and period the same way.

I was a woman who would leave for a trip to Jamaica without considering where I was in my cycle, only to bleed the moment I boarded the plane. I was a woman who stained all of her underwear and sheets with blood. I was a woman who didn't know why she briefly felt sad. Aside from complaining about my cramps, I didn't consider my period a major factor in my existence. I had a roommate who used Hormonology, an app that tracks your period, and I thought it seemed dumb. How boring! Responsible! How wretched! Denial was much more comfortable. In fact, I hated my period. I railed against it, treated it like shit, resented it. Weren't we supposed to hate it? Wasn't that why women used to call it "the curse"?

✦

I was born with a cute little cyst smack in the middle of my nose. When I was five, I was twirling in socks on a slippery, clean wooden floor at my neighbor's house and fell on my face. The cyst popped, bled, and flattened.

Then it grew back. At the doctor's office, they told us I'd have to get it removed. Otherwise it would keep growing inside of my nose and clog my nostrils. *If I don't get this cyst removed, I won't be able to breathe, and I'll die!* I remember telling girlfriends. I doubt that's how the doctor put it, but at six I was already prone to histrionics, I guess. The recovery from surgery was nice. There's a black-and-white photograph of me holding my beloved teddy bear in one hand and a balloon in another. I was given a make-your-own-chewing-gum kit and remember playing with a Cinderella sticker book.

The cysts disappeared for a few decades until I was twenty-four. Until then, all I had was a slight scar on my nose, proud of it the way most are proud of their own scars. A story you repeat to make yourself seem more interesting.

Cystic acne doesn't just mean a small under-the-skin zit. The cysts do grow under the skin, but they never come to a head like a zit does. They get as big as a quarter, under your skin, changing the entire shape and look of your face. They only express (a nicer word for "pop," or "burst pus") when they want to, and there's nothing topical to help them. They sometimes need to be drained, lanced, or shot with cortisone. (No one said this book was going to be sexy.)

The cysts were cyclical, and each time one finally expressed and flattened (and scarred), another one would appear. They became so paralyzing that I went on spironolactone, a medication originally meant for high blood pressure. Scientists realized it blocks testosterone and other androgens and could help with hormonal acne.

But I'd gone off the spironolactone because of side effects, and I was exhausted from trying to act normal while my face was bleeding and pussing and distorted. I remember one month when Tony kept asking what it was and I kept crying and then he asked if it was skin stuff and I said yes and cried myself to sleep. I had huge open wounds on the sides of my nose I made the mistake of picking at, and they wouldn't stop bleeding.

I downloaded Hormonology, but I didn't look at it for a couple months. I still thought it was dumb.

✦

When I open Hormonology now, I see that I only took notes during one month, June 2017:

> Day 20 of cycle: Moody and cranky from lack of sleep but OK. Huuuuuuuge cyst.
>
> Day 21 of cycle: Have some acne on right side of face, not sure if it's from going off of spironolactone or period. Could be worse. Feel mentally good today. Huge cyst on left side.
>
> Day 23 of cycle: Huge cystic flareup on chin.
>
> Day 26 of cycle: Cyst on cheek and picked a fight with Tony. Anxious and depressed. Incredibly huge hormonal tits.
>
> Day 1 of cycle: Miserable. Began bleeding. Cyst on left cheek. Cramps, got anxious and depressed. Picked fight with Tony.
>
> Day 2 of cycle: Still a little anxious and depressed.

Between Days 3 and 19 I didn't write anything, likely because those were the days I functioned normally.

It's funny how we don't do things we know we should do until we want to. Like how I bought Tony *Allen Carr's Easy Way to Stop Smoking* and he just put it in the back closet until he was ready, six months later.

Hormonology was created by Gabrielle Lichterman and I

ended up preferring it to all the other period trackers I'd seen my friends use, because it gave concrete tips and facts. For example: Orgasms are stronger in the days leading up to ovulation. Taking ibuprofen each morning for three days before your period will ease cramps. During the second week of your cycle, pain is blunted, so it's a good time to get bikini waxes or a tattoo. On the flip side, you're also more susceptible to getting sick during week two, while estrogen levels drop. During week four of your cycle, you are prone to negative dreams because rising progesterone makes you more prone to worry and anxiety. My favorite was Day 23, where the hormone-scope says: "Did the world and all the people in it suddenly become more annoying or is it just you? It's just you."

Female Forecaster is Hormonology's sister app, meant for the partner of the menstruating person to help prepare for their moods. FF is structured in colors: the yellow week is the happy one, the pink day is possible ovulation, green is leading up to PMS, and red is seven days of, in my case, hell on earth.

The apps were pretty sexist: for example, Female Forecaster tells the partner (which it assumes is a cis man) how high or low their menstruating partner's sex drive will be, but Hormonology *doesn't* tell the menstruating person anything along those lines.

Tony downloaded FF and put the dates of my period in his settings. Whenever I started to be symptomatic and was denying it, he would hold up his phone like a protection device, saying, "I know you're in the red zone right now! The app says I have to be strong and like a rock for you today!"

For a while, we were diligent, and I'd even write THE RED ZONE on our calendar to be prepared.

✦

In the red zone, my heart beats faster. Emotions are on speed. Whatever is in my line of vision, I have a millisecond fantasy of throwing or smashing it, and am lucky when I don't follow through. My breath is short and full of fire. I turn into a person I recognize as my *other*. My voice is higher pitched and panicked; my face wobbles with emotion and is ready to burst— usually with some inflamed under-the-skin hormonal acne in the jaw area. My eyes look smaller and sadder and the opposite of bright, and my hair is greasy and matted to my head. My body vibrates with rage.

In the red zone, I wear sweatshirts. I smell like Tiger Balm. My feet ache through the night. Once, during intense red zone rage, Tony said my eyes were fluttering and basically rolled into the back of my head.

The women in the Werewolf Week Reddit group agree:

My significant other says I get droopy eyes.

I think I look uglier and have dead skin.

I definitely get oilier!

I feel like my whole face becomes more relaxed because I can't

be bothered/don't have the energy to have facial expressions if that
makes sense. It's like even my facial muscles are done.

There's a dead-behind-the-eyes and constant vacant look.

I'm reminded of a part in the documentary about Bobby
Fischer, the chess champion, that says that people who play
chess are often in a state of doom. Because they spend so many
hours of their day thinking about how the wrong move could
take everything down, it's hard for their brain to not think that
way all the time. This is why chess players develop paranoia.
"A good player *is* paranoid on the board. When you bring that
paranoia to life, it doesn't play so well." Similarly, looking at
subjects and experiences from every possible angle serves me
when I write, and does not serve me when I am trying to move
on from an argument with Tony.

✦

In France, they use the term Zone Rouge for the areas that are
noncontiguous and deemed too damaged by conflict for human habitation.

Wikipedia says that, in football, "play while in the red zone
involves closer cramping of the offense and defense." There's a
television channel called NFL RedZone. I saw it in a commercial on a hotel television once.

Tony uses Old Spice deodorant and we noticed that at the
very top of it, it read RED ZONE COLLECTION in small letters.

Since then, though, they've redesigned, and now RED ZONE COLLECTION is written in a large, chunky font, quite similar to the font the NFL uses. I know, because I googled it.

It makes me wonder if there is something about the word "zone" that is thought of as masculine. An ex-boyfriend once told me that his ex-girlfriend would call the nights he spent alone playing video games "boy zone." In baseball, there is the strike zone.

Discovery Zone. I always wanted to go but my mom hated those places. I get it now; I hate them, too.

One humid afternoon, I took a walk to the local bookshop and café. While browsing, I came across a graphic novel of the same name as my manuscript-in-progress.

The synopsis for *The Red Zone: An Earthquake Story*: "Matteo, Guilia, and Federico have ordinary lives: they spend time with friends, help out their families, go to school, and deal with the many mood swings that come with growing up. Then, in a single night, everything changes. The ground shakes. An earthquake devastates their town and their security. But after everything is gone, life must go on. Anger and fear affect everyone in the community, but each of them must find a way to begin again. In the aftermath, the roots for stronger friendships can be laid amid the rubble."

At the end of the book, there is a note from the author.

"The story you just read is very special to me," she writes. "*The Red Zone* is a story that shows how easily the balance of our lives can be interrupted. However, we can help each other, we can stand up, we can rebuild our 'red zone.'"

✦

I was getting tired of having to rebuild our red zone. Of being damaged by conflict. The outbursts come on so quickly. Imagine a fire hydrant you're standing next to, bursting. You didn't see it coming but neither did the fire hydrant.

Now that I was tracking my period, I could see my symptoms began seven to ten days before bleeding. They occasionally ceased as soon as my period came on, and other times lasted through the first day of my period. I hoped that my tracking with my app, on our shared Google Calendar, would be enough to prevent each month from outburst and recovery.

My symptoms usually lasted ten days, then my period for five. I'd have ten days after that of normalcy, only for the symptoms to kick back in around Day 20 of the cycle. We knew the red zone came on when my thinking became cut and dried, black and white. We knew I was in the red zone when my language changed and my go-to words were "always" and "never" and "asshole." I knew I was in the red zone when I'd flip Tony off when his back was to me or he'd left the room. Later, watching the show *Divorce*, I saw Sarah Jessica Parker's character do the same thing.

✦

Tony and I needed more help than Hormonology and FF could give us, so we tried using it in conjunction with another app called The Warning: Track Her PMS. This app has you put in your period dates exactly down to the *minute*. Then it sends "the warning" to your partner's phone: *Chloe should start experiencing mood swings right now.*

One evening I was in the kitchen doing the dishes and he yelled from the living room: "What day did you get your period last month?"

"The twenty-sixth!"

"What time?"

I burst into laughter, realizing no one had ever asked me what time I'd gotten my period.

✦

A photograph of baby-pink gummies shaped like doughnuts comes up in my advertisements on Instagram. The ad claims the gummies help with mood swings, bloating, hormonal acne, and cramps. On the website is a slogan: PMS F*CKING

SUCKS. There are three women in pink towels and pink sunglasses.

I'm pretty desperate, but even *I* wouldn't purchase these so-called vitamins. They aren't even safe enough to eat on the Whole30, because they have added sugar. I mean, come on. Really? They also claim that since the gummy is strawberry-flavored and sugary, it will rid you of cravings for anything sugary, say, a brownie or a milkshake. LMAO. That said, a friend of mine swears they help her PMS, so maybe I'm jaded.

In the comments on the Instagram post, one woman wrote: "Or women could stop using their period as an excuse to be rude and hateful. (Don't come at me, I'm a woman.)"

Someone replied: "I agree with you. Nothing gives others the right to treat others like trash. I have bad hormones and rough pregnancies—doesn't mean I get to yell and scream like a banshee and hurt others. It's a matter of willpower."

Is it, though?

In 2015, my friend Diana Spechler wrote an article, "This Is My Brain on PMS," for *The New York Times*: "Most of my interpersonal conflicts happen just before my period—problems that would arise eventually anyway, but impaired by PMDD, I'm intolerant. I'm impossible. I pick fights. I jump to damaging conclusions. Maybe that's the worst of me. Or maybe that's me. Roseanne Barr once noted, 'Women complain about PMS, but I think of it as the only time of the month when I can be myself.'"

✦

Occasionally, when I'm in my good week, my golden week, around my ovulation day, I notice I get a deep yearning— deeper than one should get for something so superficial—to want to paint my nails red. Have them painted, rather.

I've had maybe six manicures in my life. Have most people had more? Less? I've always been wildly envious of women with manicures. If you have a manicure, you have to have your shit together. I've had dozens of pedicures. But my nails are not a place of beauty. They are tiny, short, ragged, and only a few times in my life have I grown them to the point that they are possible to paint. The women at the nail salons yell at me for biting them.

But in my golden week, I crave a bright red manicure. I want to look groomed. I fantasize about it—I have this idea that red will make me feel better, that red nails will give me the motivation to write, the way other people feel about red lip-stick. In her documentary, Marina Abramović says that when you're sick, if you put on a bright red outfit it helps you heal more quickly.

I don't even have a red that I go to. I stare at oranges, pinks, rusts, seafoam greens, grays for way too long, embarrassingly long. I forget that I'm not choosing my fate, just a dumbass color no one will care about or notice. But I love reading the bottom of the bottles, the names. Cha-ching Cherry. Rebel Fox. Rouge Rubis. Lover. Red Silk Boxers. It's Raining Men.

Tomorrow's Red. Rouge Puissant. Candy Apple. Pirate. Sensation. Black Cherry. Single Ladies. Gangsta Boo. Red Silk Boxers. Limited Addiction. I grab a random red.

After my nails are painted, I feel powerful. I type and I do the dishes and stroke my partner's skin, and I look like I have different hands.

A week goes by, I don't bite my nails, I feel good about my appearance. But then I hit the red zone and my personality flips. I am anxious, worried. Tony says he can see in my eyes I don't think he loves me. I drink a few glasses of wine and sit in the dark on the sweet little yellow couch we bought together last spring. I start with one nail, promising myself I will leave the rest alone. Then I peel another off, make the promise again, and this goes on—this making and breaking of promises, until all the nail polish, the polish that has loved me so well, is left chipped on my fingers (which some people can pull off really well, let's admit it), and in the morning when I wake up and go to the yellow couch, I see the small, sad pile, the remnants, the proof of how I felt the previous night, on the couch.

I clean them up and throw them in the garbage, knowing the red-nail-polish-turned-nail-biting cycle will repeat in another month or two.

THE CYCLE

The Golden Week

A picnic at Shakespeare & Company in Lenox, Massachusetts. We were constantly buying picnic baskets. We were really into liver pâté from a local shop in our town. Olives stuffed with garlic. One weekend, high on dopamine, we bought small yellow bunny cups and plates. "I will protect your heart," we said to each other.

{Ovulation}

The Red Zone

In the beginning, the outbursts were almost always about a woman.

Tony came back to town to visit for a weekend before his next week in Fire Island for work. He brought back a beautiful black dress and a pair of earrings for me. I'd spent the day alone in manic love with him while he was at a wedding, playing piano. I had a cyst coming on and was reading on Reddit that the best way to get them to disappear is putting rice into a clean sock, tying the sock closed, heating the sock up in the microwave, and holding the rice-filled sock to your face, repeating this when the sock loses heat. It's supposed to help the blood spread out, move the pus on the inside around. Problem is, I didn't have a microwave. I did it anyway, by holding the sock against my boiling teakettle, then holding it to my cheek. For hours I stood in the kitchen doing this while reading student essays and marking them with a red pen. I called my mom and told her about the sock trick. "Just make sure the sock is clean," she said.

I was in a good mood, feeling so lucky to be dating such a thoughtful person. When Tony arrived back at my apartment, though, he said he had to check on his Airbnbers, three women who were staying at his place while he stayed at mine. They were at a local bar, and he wanted to swing by with me to say hello.

Instant rage. I interpreted this as the rudest possible thing anyone could ever do to me.

"I feel rejected, humiliated, and rejected!"

I stormed out, slamming my door (I pity the new tenant who lived below me, as slamming doors was my signature move in those days) and began walking down the street toward the river. Tony followed behind me. He was like, "Do you really think I want to go fuck three of my Airbnb guests? What the hell are you talking about?"

As time went on and we kept airbnbing, I learned Tony was a Superhost and held on to that status like it was gold, which it was. One of the ways he kept the status up was by greeting and talking with all his guests.

The Repair

Of course in the morning I began bleeding. We went to the grocery store so Tony could get some groceries to bring with him back to Fire Island. He had one more week of work and had driven all the way back upstate just to spend a night together. Cue my remorse. We went to brunch on a patio and discussed how to handle misunderstandings better in the future. A lot of our fights revolved around the shared Airbnb calendar and Airbnb miscommunications. We decided he'd share the Airbnb calendar with me so I'd know when he had guests, and therefore would be sleeping at my place.

The Golden Week

Sadie was turning seven and Tony wanted to take her to Legoland for her birthday. I still didn't know how many of their activities to join and when to give them space. Tony wanted me to come, but I made sure he asked first. I heard him say to

Sadie, "When we go to Legoland, do you want to go you and me, or you, me, and Chloe?"

"You me and Chloe," she responded.

We drove to Legoland playing games in the car. She liked the one where we had to find words on signs in the order of the alphabet as we drove. She liked when I drew on her arm with my finger so she could guess what I was writing. "It tickles!" she said.

Tony had Airbnbers at his apartment so they slept over, Sadie on my pull-out futon in the living room. In the morning, she created a Legoland in my living room. We drove to McDonald's because she'd never had a Happy Meal before.

{Ovulation}

The Red Zone

I'd accidentally spilled a glass of water onto my laptop and texted Tony that I was going to throw it out my kitchen window, into an alley. He came over. I told him not to.

"What did you do immediately after you spilled a glass of water on it?"

"I took a bath. Then I plugged it in."

"Plugging it in is the first thing it says *not* to do, if you google it."

"I didn't give a fuck about googling it. I wanted to take a bath and chuck it in the alley."

He held his head in his hands, laughing, frustrated. I told him to leave.

The Repair

We'd laugh about these mishaps, outbursts, dramas, when my sense of humor returned. I kept thinking that since I was aware of the cycle I'd be able to control it next time.

In *Abandon Me*, Melissa Febos writes: "Self-knowledge didn't save you, it only made it hurt more to watch yourself."

A decade ago my mom had told me not to pick fights just to make up, or test someone. For me, it wasn't that at all. God, how badly I didn't want to fight. I remember wishing I could pay a sum of money to someone to make the outbursts stop. I remember praying to a period god I wasn't sure existed to make it stop, to *please* make it stop.

The Golden Week

We walked holding hands to the local hardware store to make apartment keys for each other. The man asked if we wanted them in silver or gold. "Gold," we said in unison. We went to dinner that night and accidentally ordered a large sea bass (we thought we'd ordered the small one) and then the doggy bag went back and forth between our apartments.

{Ovulation}

The Red Zone

Tony was in Denver for work and had traveled to Boulder for the weekend to visit friends. He was having dinner with his friend Keith from music school and his friend's family.

On the phone, Tony relayed a detail about Keith's wife's plans to be out of town. But it sounded as if she actually was in town. This could not be more irrelevant, but during the red zone, irrelevant details become important to fixate on.

I said, "I thought you said his wife wasn't going to be there."

"She is here," he acknowledged.

"I know. Why did you say she wasn't going to be?"

I don't know why I cared about this. I did not know Tony's friend, or his wife, and it truly didn't affect anything. My heart was on fire and my hands were shaking. I knew I was being fucked with. I paced my apartment. Breathing fire.

That's when an eight-second audio message came in. Tony and I send audio messages to each other all day, so this was not out of the ordinary. But when I hit play I heard hearty laughter. In one full breath he said, "Oh my god women are so fucking hilarious."

He had accidentally recorded a voice memo and sent it, so I received this gem of a snippet. The fact that it wasn't meant for my ears made it sting.

I flipped the fuck out. Hard. I called him a douchebag. I said I always knew he was a dick. I thought we were friends!

"I'm *all* women now?! I'm your employee? Ex-wife? Daughter? How the fuck are you going to categorize me as *all women*?!?!?!"

I'd imagined Tony sitting at a dinner party, laughing at my text and sharing it with everyone.

Tony's version: He was alone walking to Keith's car. Keith was already in the car and they were about to drive to a liquor store. They'd just eaten dinner with Keith, Keith's wife, Keith's mom, Keith's two daughters, and Keith's wife's friend. His release of "ohmygodwomenaresofuckinghilarious" was born from that. It is true that when I listened to the message again, I could hear that he was laughing alone. It is also true that I was being fucking hilarious.

While Keith went into the liquor store, Tony called to talk me off the ledge, which took about an hour.

Instead of calling me a bitch or something like that, he moved toward kindness. "I understand that, *sweetheart*," he said, in place of "psycho."

The next day I woke up bleeding, and the day after that, I treasured that voice message.

"Wow, that did a real one-eighty," Tony said.

Over the next week, when I'd calmed down, I forwarded the voice memo to a bunch of my friends. Everyone loved it. When we feel batshit, we begin texting each other: OMG WOMEN ARE SO FUCKING HILARIOUS.

He is so lucky the adjective he'd chosen was *hilarious*. He could have said: ridiculous. Annoying. Insane. Imagine if he had said, "Women are so fucking crazy."

"Do you like fighting?" he asked me from time to time. "You must really love arguing," he'd say.

"No. I just come from fighting."

I remember my boobs were the biggest they'd ever been from bloating.

The Repair

Anna, my therapist, talked about how I knew how to *kill with words*. I loved shooting off text messages to get a sense of power. *Reckless speaking.* She told me I could begin to say, "I could eviscerate you with words right now, but I'm not going to."

The Golden Week

I'd wake up with a feeling of *Look what I got!* I had hearts in my eyes, like a cartoon character. *Look what I got!* I felt I was saying to the baristas, bartenders, and library clerks. *Can you believe I got this?* I was almost embarrassed by the fact that I'd so obviously gotten what I never admitted, nor known, I'd wanted. Sadie and I bonded over Tony's sleeptalking, which I'd hear at night and write into the Notes app on my phone. She'd beg me to record it each night and show it to her in the morning.

"I'm never ordering exotic animals off Craigslist again" was one of his most famous lines. Another time he said, "No. I'm not buying that banana for you."

"Why?" I asked.

"Because it's old, it's brown, and all you can do with it as this point is use it as phone."

{Ovulation}

The Red Zone

Tony was directing an opera and had needed a specific spiral binding to hold the music score. He only needed two but could only bulk order a hundred. They arrived in a huge cardboard box. He was already stressed out and annoyed about the box and in a fit of frustrated rage kicked it down the stairs. The small metal spirals took up residence there for the night.

The Repair

If you think this is one of those books where the woman is batshit and her partner is a rock, it isn't. Tony was by no means just a steady silent type. Though I am the villain in this memoir, Tony had *stuff*, too. At thirty-seven, he had already been through the wringer. Of course he was reactive to my energy in the red zone, and would also yell and become riled up, condescend and provoke. I've struggled with this paragraph in every draft of the book, and have even tried listing his flaws and faults here, but it felt cheap. He had his own issues; they just weren't severe PMS.

When I told Anna we'd met and were dating I was self-righteously going off, saying, "I was supposed to stay single and pave the way for other women, and all of my students!"

"Sounds like he's really fucking up your plan," she joked.

She said, "You're both on the same path." She gave us both a copy of *Transforming Relationships: Come as You Are* by David R. Gilroy and Donna R. Baker-Gilroy. It was "a psycho-spiritual guide for couples that maps the path from conflict to peace." It provides a guide for living relationships with acceptance, compassion, and authenticity rather than having to give up or change who you really are.

Sometimes after a fight we'd meditate together in the morning. We'd go to brunch and drink coffee with cinnamon over Dutch baby pancakes.

The Red Zone

My landlady sent me a text message with a couple of aggressive exclamation points and capitalizations referring to a misunderstanding over a utility bill, and I ended up enraged and screaming for roughly forty-five minutes. Tony was at the ocean on Fire Island working for a nonprofit dance company. When I called, he'd been swimming and laughing in the waves of the ocean, he later told me. Then I called. Our conversation:

"I just want you to agree with me that she's a bitch," I said.

"I am agreeing with you," he replied.

"No, you're appeasing me."

This went on and escalated for fifteen minutes until: *"Jesus Christ,* Chloe, what does your heart need?"

"I need you to agree with me."

"I am agreeing with you. "

"No, you aren't, not wholeheartedly."

After we got off the phone, I brought it back up over text, and I had to bring it up the day after that, too. I was stuck. I could not let those exclamation points go. I could not fathom anyone seeing this situation in any other way than how I saw it. I swore and berated via text. My fingers kept flying.

✦

We were out to breakfast and I ordered a coffee with half-and-half like a normal person. The waiter scoffed at me: "We don't use *half-and-half* here."

Tony said, "Yeah I've been getting almond milk in my cappuccinos."

"I love half-and-half," I said.

"Well, soon you won't." She eyed me. "It'll catch up with you."

Enraged. How dare not one but *two* people shame me for using half-and-half? You talk shit about half-and-half and you're talking shit about me and my family. There are photos of my dad back in the eighties when I was born and he had a rattail and there is a purple carton of Hood half-and-half in the background. Both my parents still use it. My cousin used to drink the small ones they give out at diners and I thought she was the coolest person in the world for doing so. Half-and-half is in my bloodstream and it is the only way my coffee will turn the color I want it to. Plus, it's fucking delicious. Ever had a breve?

I left breakfast and walked home, seething. When I am in this mode, I take action; it is hard to stay still.

Tony caught up to me before we'd made it back to the apartment. "Kiss me, you *fuck*," he said, and we did, then walked back to breakfast. We checked the app and realized my period was at least three weeks away, and that I wasn't even in the red zone yet. I was in the week between golden and red.

"Fuck," he said. "So, it can even happen in any zone?"

"Yeah that wasn't the red zone," I said. "That was just my personality."

✦

When I ask Tony now how he dealt with this season of our lives, he tells me it was because he played the long game. Back then, I could only see a couple days ahead. But he saw things differently, wasn't as caught up in the day-to-day, and I think that's because he's been married before and has a daughter.

He saw the big picture. I had tunnel vision. We even have different mindsets when it comes to toilet paper; he will buy huge packages to last months, whereas I will only buy one roll at a time.

DARK MATTER

My doctor looked like my ninth grade biology teacher, who always ground my gears. She had us dissect a pig, and over fifteen years later, I could remember the smell of pig juices and blood. The class was in the morning. It would have been a better life skill if she'd had us dissect a uterus.

Through my twenties I didn't have a doctor or health insurance so the whole sterile environment was new for me. Now I use Medicaid. If I had a high co-pay and had to shell out hundreds of dollars for medication, I wouldn't be able to experiment this way.

It hadn't occurred to me to check with Tony before I got on board with taking antidepressants. But when I told him, he was concerned I wouldn't be able to sleep well, eat well, or orgasm well. "Those are the fun parts of life," he said.

He'd said he could handle my massive mood swings. He'd said that I was basing our relationship on just two days a month, even though it was great the rest of the time. That's the frustrating thing. PMDD can kick in any time after the day you ovulate. This means that for fourteen days until your period, it's all up in the air.

But *I* couldn't handle them. And I knew that after some time he wouldn't be able to anymore. The decision to finally try medication was one based in fear—fear of losing the love I'd found.

Somehow I had the foresight to record the conversation with my doctor-who-looked-like-my-biology-teacher on my phone because I thought it'd be funny to listen to later. As it turned out, it was just kind of sad: the dismissiveness, the lack of interest and even deeper lack of knowledge.

The voice memo from September 2017:

"What brings you in?"

"My period," I say, and then speak for almost another three minutes. In one breath I say: "Leading up to my period first I get a cyst, I get really bad leg cramps, a headache, then I have what to me feels like an episode where I scream. And cry. About the tiniest thing. There's a sense of mania to it—I can feel great and then I'm *shaking* I'm so mad with rage, angry, sad, and go to a really dark place."

I remember her nodding vacantly. On the recording she says: "So, irritability."

Not exactly. It's like how in the film *The Story of Menstru-ation*, released by Disney in 1946, they describe premenstrual syndrome as: "Some girls have a little less pep." Yeah, that's one way to put it.

The doctor wrote me a prescription for Zoloft. Why Zoloft? She had zero reasons to back her up. Whenever I asked her any questions, she made a generalization or said, "I don't know."

I was desperate, though, and in tears, and happily accepted.

I was instructed to take half a blue pill of Zoloft each day of the month until the week leading up to my period when I was supposed to take a full pill, beginning on the day I ovulated.

◆

I'd been on the Zoloft a couple weeks when I went down to New York to attend the Franklin Park Reading Series in Crown Heights, Brooklyn. It was my first day of taking a full pill. The September weather in the city was perfect and hopeful. I sat at the bar and chose a fruit-flavored beer.

Friends showed up and we all sat in a booth. Someone took a photo of us that three out of four of us ended up posting on Instagram. We put in an order for burgers and fries. I looked at my phone and had a text from Tony: "You have a very interesting way of cutting avocados."

Uzodinma and Elizabeth were talking near the room with the bar games, and Elizabeth motioned for me to come chat with them.

I walked over, then became violently nauseated, sweating profusely, staring at Uzodinma's braces while I spoke, realizing

I'd have to run past him to get to the bathroom to vomit. Then
I blacked out.

Over email, Uzodinma gave me his version of what had
happened.

> I had to kind of squat down and deadlift you
> under the arms. I tried to lift you onto my
> shoulder but couldn't do it. I decided to try
> and get you over to a chair, as opposed to let-
> ting you crumple in a heap on the floor. The
> bouncer came over and was just watching me.
> I'm having this totally insane conversation/
> argument trying to get him to help me get
> you over to a chair or one of the benches. I
> think he thought I was on some Bill Cosby
> shit or something. Everyone in that area,
> now, is watching, trying to figure out what's
> going on. He's just standing there staring at
> me, my arms give out, I try to at least ease you
> down, keep you from getting hurt, and right
> after that you woke up . . .

Uzodinma said I looked up at him from the floor and said,
"I'm on antidepressants." He told me later that he'd thought I
was making a joke.

Apparently I stood back up, and then fainted again, caught

by Elizabeth and Uzodinma. I was unconscious for another minute. When I woke up again, I was drenched in sweat. The bar was dark and I hoped people just thought I was crouched down getting something out of my purse. The bouncer was next to me, on the phone with 911.

I panicked. My narrative about myself is that I have no health problems. I never used to take medication; I've never broken a bone or even sprained a joint, never spent a night in a hospital. I'm not even allergic to anything. At my doctor's appointments, it often felt gloat-worthy the way my forms always read *no no no no no*. No, I don't have this, or that. I always felt I impressed doctors, and loved when they'd make an insinuation that I was very healthy, and easy.

But now the ambulance was on its way. I went outside with Uzodinma and Elizabeth and brought my burger. Meanwhile, the people on the phone (911?) with the bouncer were telling him to tell me *not* to eat, and I wasn't taking this news well. Elizabeth later imitated my crying about my burger.

"I think you should let her eat the fucking burger, *man*," Uzodinma said, a statement I am eternally grateful for. The bouncer finally agreed. I took a bite of the burger and it was dry as fuck.

Elizabeth climbed into the ambulance with me, wearing black stilettos. A bunch of other writer acquaintances showed up with concern on their faces. I asked Elizabeth to tell them to go away. All the attention and "What's wrong?" inquiries when *I* didn't know what was wrong scared me, and I was embarrassed to be causing such a scene.

The woman took my blood pressure and it was low. I told her I'd recently gotten blood tests back and was anemic.

"Me, too!" she said. "Eat more bloody steak."

They asked me multiple times if I wanted to go to the emergency room and I declined.

I left without saying goodbye to anyone. I walked to the 5 train, then took the 1 train to the Amtrak station, and arrived in Hudson two hours later. I walked back to Tony's, the same place I'd started the day. In bed I received an email from Uzodinma with the subject line *9/11*, which was the date. *You get home OK?* he asked. *Shit got crazy there for a second.*

The irony that the tiny blue pill I'd taken to *stabilize* my moods led to me sobbing in an ambulance was not lost on anyone. Tony and I laughed about it that night, considering how irresponsible my drinking and drug habits have been in the past, and how none of it had ever made me faint or landed me in an ambulance. Then I take a Zoloft and black the fuck out. What the actual hell?

✦

I'd tried meds and failed. Not only failed but fainted in public. Medication didn't like me, and I didn't like it, either. I was discouraged. Back to being hopeless. I threw away the Zoloft.

✦

I muscled through a few months without meds, but it all came to a head in December, and I flipped shit at the American Museum of Natural History.

I'd woken up that Friday with my period and was ecstatic that I hadn't had too bad of an outburst. I'd almost had two the previous week—one where I invented the idea that Tony didn't care I was sick (I wasn't that sick) and another where we had a miscommunication about making chili. We got through both incidents in just an hour and there were no tears.

I had slept at the Jane Hotel with my friend Eliza, who was visiting from Tucson, Arizona. When I told Eliza I was afraid of my period, and asked her about hers, she said the only thing that happened when she got her period was a light twinge in her abdomen. I was jealous.

"You'll be okay," she said.

"Probably not," I responded, packing THC salve and ibuprofen into my bag.

We walked to the Waverly Diner to meet Sadie and Tony to spend the day together before we all went back to Hudson. I ate eggs and felt happy and when we left the diner, I made a comment about the way to go to the museum. Tony told me I was wrong, pulled out his map, and showed me why. When we went underground to get the subway, I felt rage. I walked away from everyone brimming with tears. Eliza asked me, "What happened?" and I said something about Tony being an asshole, which was my absolute favorite PMDD word.

At the museum I noticed that I crumpled up my ticket in the coat of my pocket. My hand was balled in a fist and sweaty. I was embarrassed each time we went to a new thing and I had to pull my shredded and wet ticket out.

I was so enraged at Tony I could not look at him. I stopped making eye contact with him and completely ignored him—something I'd never done before. I went and sat by myself below some dinosaur skeleton. I heard Sadie ask where I was, and she came and sat with me. She was, at that point, the only person I could stand.

In the butterfly conservatory, I watched the metallic butterflies and couldn't decide if I loved or hated them. When we walked in it was humid and everyone was told to take off their scarves and coats, but the temperature suited me fine. What was my problem? Why was my body temperature different from the norm?

In line for a movie titled *Dark Universe* narrated by Neil deGrasse Tyson, I continued to talk to Eliza and to ignore Tony. The movie began and there were sparkles of pink and blue falling over us. I could not retain one fact.

Tony leaned over and began speaking to me sternly. He wanted to have a good day with his daughter. Was I able to have a good day? When he spoke this way, it made me cry. I felt so guilty, so shitty, so mad at myself, and yet could not stop. I was completely raw and enraged. Tyson's voice merged into the episode I was having; I can still hear him today.

Toward the end of the film I repeated to myself *Take his hand take his hand take his hand* and then did. I hoped I would soften, but I was so far gone. I'd come back to myself for twenty minutes, but then the wave of PMDD would hit and take me under. Boogie boarding.

My reality was not matching anyone else's. I did not feel real in my body. I texted him, "Let's just break up then."

On the Amtrak home, I sat alone by the window, with Eliza across the aisle.

That night, Tony and I slept in the guest room because Sadie fell asleep in his bed. We slept differently than usual. We stayed on one side of the bed, and he never turned away from me, not once, only toward me.

In the morning, I felt like I'd been through a mental war. Whenever the dysphoria lifts, there is a fleeting feeling of being high and light. My friend Elizabeth says the same thing happens to her after she gets through a migraine.

I wanted everything to go back to normal: to be forgiven, go back in time. I couldn't, and I knew if things continued this way, I would ruin my relationship. I was always sorry, so sorry, so sorry, and I was sick of it. Tony told me he couldn't live this way anymore.

✦

A couple months later, Tony and I were on a date at a restaurant called Rouge in West Stockbridge, Massachusetts. After our dinner, we were going to see the Ruth Bader Ginsburg movie. I was drinking a cocktail.

I told Tony I felt weird.

"I know," he said.

"I'm going to the car," I said, feeling queasy.

I woke up on the floor of the restaurant. Again.

"Do you watch *Nurse Jackie?*" I asked the woman with short blond hair who was leaning over me.

She laughed. "It's funny you say that because I'm actually a nurse," she said. She was warm and caring and I wanted her to lean over me forever.

The ambulance came. This time, I didn't get into it. The paramedics told us to go buy some liver or pâté, as that would get iron into my system the quickest. There wasn't anywhere to buy pâté or liver, so we went to the Dairy Queen drive-through and I pounded a junk food cheeseburger.

I realized that each time I've fainted it was the week after my period, after all the blood loss. I began taking iron supplements and eating chicken liver pâté again.

✦

At the American Museum of Natural History, we'd had our photo taken before going into the exhibit, with one of those fake backgrounds of dinosaurs. In the photograph, I'm grinning in between Eliza and Sadie, in a plaid scarf, a fresh haircut. Tony's smiling big, too, but probably he was braced. You wouldn't know from the photo that anything was going on internally. They sold us the photograph in a Christmas ornament, and every Christmas it appears, haunting me. We laugh when we look at it now, my psychotic grin and the gleam in my eye. Once Tony offered to throw it away, but I wanted to keep it.

PREMENSTRUAL DYSPHORIC DISORDER

When was the first time I heard of it? I'm pretty sure it was my therapist, Anna, who first said the acronym PMDD to me. I do remember having a flicker of recognition, as though I'd read about PMDD somewhere in passing.

When I got back to my apartment, I began researching.

✦

From the International Association for Premenstrual Disorders: "Premenstrual Dysphoric Disorder (PMDD) is a cyclical, hormone-based mood disorder with symptoms arising during the premenstrual or luteal phase of the menstrual cycle and subsiding within a few days of menstruation. It affects an estimated 5.5% of women and AFAB individuals of reproductive age."

Though some people who menstruate have PMDD from very young, for most it arrives at "reproductive age." I was thirty-one.

✦

I knew I'd never felt this way until now—I'd had PMS bouts, sure, but nothing like these episodes. Having a witness changed everything. Had I actually had PMDD in my twenties and just hadn't had a mirror for it? Or had it developed when I turned thirty? Or worsened because I was at reproductive age? What came first, the chicken, or the PMDD egg?

One evening Tony and I glanced through my book *Women*, and he said, "This book is riddled with PMDD." Maybe. Maybe not. Or maybe I did occasionally experience it and thought it was something else. Even more, I wonder if some of the other stuff I was doing, like yoga teacher training or acupuncture or trying a supplement or herbs, or even good old-fashioned drugs, eradicated it, numbed it, or supported it. I'll never know, and I won't pretend to know, either. What I know: what I began experiencing in my thirties I had never experienced before.

✦

PMDD was added to the list of depressive disorders in the *Diagnostic and Statistical Manual of Mental Disorders* in 2013. There are eleven possible symptoms, and, according to Wikipedia, a person has to exhibit a minimum of five symptoms in order to qualify for PMDD. To *qualify*. I love how this was phrased like a challenge, like having to be tall enough to go on a certain ride at Disneyland.

To be diagnosed, your symptoms also must correlate with your menstrual cycle. During the follicular phase of your cycle, PMDD sufferers' symptoms cease. Post-ovulation, symptoms continually become worse, until the onset of bleeding.

The diagnostic criteria, according to the DSM:

Timing of symptoms

A. In the majority of menstrual cycles, at least 5 symptoms must be present in the final week before the onset of menses, start to improve within a few days after the onset of menses, and become minimal or absent in the week postmenses

Symptoms

B. One or more of the following symptoms must be present:
  1) Marked affective lability (e.g., mood swings, feeling suddenly sad or tearful, or increased sensitivity to rejection)
  2) Marked irritability or anger or increased interpersonal conflicts

3) Markedly depressed mood, feelings
of hopelessness, or self-deprecating
thoughts

4) Marked anxiety, tension, and/or feelings of being keyed up or on edge

C. One (or more) of the following symptoms
must additionally be present to reach a
total of 5 symptoms when combined with
symptoms from criterion B above:

1) Decreased interest in usual activities

2) Subjective difficulty in concentration

3) Lethargy, easy fatigability, or marked
lack of energy

4) Marked change in appetite; overeat-
ing or specific food cravings

5) Hypersomnia or insomnia

6) A sense of being overwhelmed or out
of control

7) Physical symptoms such as breast
tenderness or swelling; joint or mus-
cle pain; a sensation of "bloating" or
weight gain

Severity

D. The symptoms are associated with clini-
cally significant distress or interference

with work, school, usual social activities,
or relationships with others.

E. Consider Other Psychiatric Disorders:
The disturbance is not merely an exacerbation of the symptoms of another disorder, such as major depressive disorder,
panic disorder, persistent depressive disorder (dysthymia) or a personality disorder (although it may co-occur with any of
these disorders).

Confirmation of the disorder

F. Criterion A should be confirmed by pro-
spective daily ratings during at least 2
symptomatic cycles (although a provi-
sional diagnosis may be made prior to this
confirmation)

Exclude Other Medical Explanations

G. The symptoms are not attributable to the
physiological effects of a substance (e.g.,
drug abuse, medication or other treatment) or another medical condition (e.g.,
hyperthyroidism).

Women are often misdiagnosed with bipolar disorder, schizo-phrenia, and major depressive disorder, which doctors seem to go to before looking at the menstrual cycle.

Here's one image that has stuck with me—a photograph with a split screen: one side reads *PMS* with a photo of a woman pulling her hair out, and the other side reads *PMDD* with a woman on the edge of a rooftop.

"Have you had any freak-outs on Tony recently?" my friend Hannah asked me. I told her I had. I asked her if she'd ever had those pre-period.

"Yeah, I mean I think I had one on you the last time we hung out."

She had. We'd been in my apartment on a sunny afternoon and she'd left, screaming that I was a selfish bitch. Later she texted that she'd been feeling hormonal. I'd never had a fight to that extent with her and was shaken up afterward, so I had a tiny bit of experience being on the other side.

✦

When PMDD originally hit the scene, some feminists were angry. Some feminist psychologists believed that the language surrounding PMDD is misleading and that its classification as a psychiatric disorder stigmatizes women as mentally ill and covers up the real reasons for women's anguish. "It's a label that can be used by a sexist society that wants to believe that many women go crazy once a month," Paula J. Caplan, PhD, author of *They Say You're Crazy*, explains.

But Joan C. Chrisler, PhD, a psychology professor at Connecticut College and president of the Society for Menstrual Cycle Research, counters by saying the most important thing is to give women who seek help validation. "Whatever they're experiencing, they're experiencing."

I'd gone to a dinner with some acquaintances a few months after learning what PMDD was, and as I confided in them what I was experiencing, one person pushed back, saying PMDD didn't exist; your body was doing what it was supposed to be doing and the label was bullshit, a way to hold women back, patriarchal and misogynistic.

I said it was nice to have a name for it.

She said, "If you have to call it something, call it Jason."

Though it was hurtful to be thought of—by another woman especially—as being dramatic or making it all up, my mission wasn't to convince anyone of anything. I'm not going to pretend I know exactly how PMDD works; I only know how it *feels*. It is a mystery, and the studies around it have continually developed and changed over the five years of writing this book.

Dysphoria is Greek for *difficult to bear*. WebMD says: "Dysphoria: a profound state of unease and dissatisfaction. In a psychiatric context, dysphoria may accompany depression, anxiety, or agitation. It can also refer to a state of not being comfortable in one's current body. The opposite state of mind is known as euphoria."

I certainly know what euphoria feels like, as I've taken a small share of MDMA in my day. When I'm in euphoria, I have felt beautiful, compassionate to my acne scars, one with the world. I have felt . . . *sparkly*. Now I knew what the opposite felt like, too.

✦

On *Salon*, I read an article called "The real Sylvia Plath." It argues that Plath perhaps didn't suffer from manic depression, but from severe PMS. It suggests that the poems in her book *Ariel*, published in 1965, were not just figurative, abstract expressions of Plath's preoccupation with female fertility, but were directly correlated with Plath's biology. "Metaphors for ovulation and menstrual blood are prevalent in her late work," says Katherine Dalton, a PMS researcher.

Ariel. My brother gave me that book for my eighteenth birthday. I turned to my right, my bookshelf, and saw it sitting directly across from me, as if it had been waiting for the past sixteen years for me to notice it. Inside it was inscribed: READ IT. LOVE IT. 2004.

I began scouring it for signs of PMDD. The word "blood" was on almost every other page. I also found embryos, blood clots, roses, wombs, babies, pink, red lions, bloody skirts.

✦

I became an amateur detective about everything: Once I went into the kitchen and asked Tony if he'd had diarrhea at all the week before. I had it on a Sunday, and it was the Saturday after. I was trying to figure out if it was a meal we'd eaten or the new magnesium supplements I'd been popping three of a day after being told they'd help my mood and cramps. I'd gotten the craziest most liquid-y diarrhea of my life.

I'd spent forty-five minutes reading Reddit and suspected it was the magnesium that was giving me the horrendous diarrhea. I'd bought magnesium citrate instead of malate. Apparently, malate is the one that's supposed to make you feel chill and citrate is the one that will give you diarrhea.

"I don't know," he said, shaking his head and getting the supplies to make more coffee. "Some are good and some are bad. I don't pay much attention to it." That is the difference between cis men and cis women: cis women will figure out where their diarrhea is coming from. Cis men won't.

✦

In 2017, when I was diagnosed, there were about three PMDD Instagram accounts. Now there are hundreds. @pmddleveluptolevelout (which began posting in 2019) writes: *PMDD Describe it in 3 Words.* The responses roll in:

Unpredictable. Terrifying. Crippling.

Debilitating mental torture.

Exhaustion. Chaos. Patience.

Hell on earth.

Vulnerability. Dangerous. Exhausting.

I relate to Ayelet Waldman and her book *A Really Good Day: How Microdosing Made a Mega Difference in My Mood, My Marriage, and My Life*: "For as long as I can remember, I have been held hostage by the vagaries of mood. . . . My symptoms have never been serious enough to require hospitalization, nor have they ever prevented me from functioning either personally or professionally, but they have made my life and the lives of the people whom I love much more difficult."

I read the book *WomanCode* by Alisa Vitti, and felt kinship with the chapter "When Bad Hormones Happen to Good Women."

Monarch butterflies are hormonal, too. Every major activity that occurs in their lives is governed by hormones. From an article in *The New York Times*: "The endocrinologist is at present seeking further hormonal explanations for the monarch's bursts of reproductive activity, which suddenly shuts down when the flashy black-and-orange insects start feeding frantically in preparation for their long flight south . . . A moth or butterfly will remain a caterpillar forever unless juvenile hormone production ceases."

Maybe PMDD is payback. Payback for wanting to be in an altered state for 75 percent of my teenage years and my twenties. I've always had a strong mind. I liked challenging that mind. The challenge of being stoned in environments you shouldn't be stoned in. The challenge of going to the waitressing job after being up all night. The challenge of doing mundane tasks on heavy drugs. Karma of the body—is that a thing?

My friend Fran has a theory that your body starts to hate you in your early thirties if you want a baby and don't have one. It can feel it. This is why, she thinks, PMDD appears at the child-rearing age.

I wonder, too, if PMDD can run in the family. After I went on a podcast to talk about PMDD, one of my cousins emailed me after having listened:

"I am shook. I cried with compassion and understanding and just a simple feeling of realization. Just last Thursday night into Friday I went through what I now truly believe was a PMDD 'episode.' Panic and paranoia and I just took myself to 'crazy town.' Such an unreal experience. This was actually one of the most real-feeling episodes I've had, and it just shook me to my core. I completely identify with what you said about the fact that at the time of an 'episode' the feeling in my body and in my heart is the realest thing I've ever felt. And then it just subsides and I confuse the shit out of myself thinking, 'Was that real? Where did those thoughts come from? Am I crazy?' After doing some more research about PMDD, I am now quite certain I have been affected by it for many years and was so totally unaware, and just suffering through—thinking I was just 'part-time crazy.' Thinking I just had depression, or was bipolar. So many diagnoses by so many therapists that didn't seem to 100 percent fit."

✦

In 1994, the film *Tom and Viv*, based on T. S. Eliot and his wife Vivienne Haigh-Wood Eliot, was released. The voice-over at the start of the film says: "Vivienne suffered from what we used to call women's troubles.

"While she occasionally acts as a muse for the poet, her inconsistent behavior may prove too much for him to bear. Her doctor diagnoses a mental disorder that leads to 'disregard for propriety.'"

Vivienne's Wikipedia page says: "She was also plagued by heavy, irregular menstruation, to her great embarrassment, and severe premenstrual tension, which led to mood swings, fainting spells, and migraines . . . She apparently felt unable to ask her mother for help. Eventually her mother took her to a doctor who prescribed potassium bromide to sedate her, which probably meant he had diagnosed 'hysteria,'" a common label for difficult women. Her Wikipedia page also claims that her marriage worsened her symptoms.

✦

In the midst of a brutal period, I walked to my friend Hannah's house to meet her five-day-old newborn. Before that, I'd been on the toilet text-fighting with Tony. "I feel zero connection to you," I'd written. "I feel rage."

"I can't control the amount of rage you feel toward me," he'd written back.

"This is the best thing to do on your period," I said, when I arrived at Hannah's. "Hold a newborn." Her husband laughed.

"You're the second person here with their period," Kaya said. "Lucy was holding the baby, and when she went to the bathroom, she saw she'd bled all over her shorts."

Sadie had a birthday party to go to at a trampoline park last weekend. Afterward, we drove past Ocean State Job Lot and bought a bunch of random shit like yogurt-covered cranberries and almonds. Sadie and I got Softlips lip balm, which she was very intrigued by after I explained that Softlips was very coveted back when I was a preteen. Tony bought me a mixed box of pads and tampons. Later Sadie asked what a tampon was and I said women use them for their period when they're older and she asked no more questions. Usually she pushes harder. I wonder if deep down she knows something scary is coming. It's unbelievable for me to remember a time I didn't know this was coming. Sometimes I wonder if that was the best part of my life.

Once you know what tampons are, you can't unknow it. I tell my students the same thing; publishing is like sex, once you do it, there's no going back. Treasure the sacred time you are unpublished and don't know what tampons are.

✦

Anna told me that my period was possibly worse every other month because we have one ovary that is more adverse than the other. One evil ovary. That's why hormonal breakouts, in my case cysts, often occur on one side of your face more than the other each month. I've learned to dread every other period and #notallperiods.

She noticed that whenever I talked about PMDD, I referred to it as "it." As though it wasn't me but another entity. I did the same thing when speaking about my acne or cysts. "My skin." Anna was big on saying no feeling is wrong, and supported me in trying to make space for all the rage. She wanted me to try integrating PMDD into who I was, instead of compartmentalizing.

On the *Armchair Expert* podcast, Dax Shepard interviewed comedian and actor Bill Hader, and the conversation turned to Hader's anxiety. He described having a panic attack on *Saturday Night Live*, the night that Jeff Bridges was hosting. After the show, Jeff Bridges went up to Hader and said, about the anxiety, "That's your buddy. Put your arm

around it. The more you battle it the more it will fight you."
Put your arm around it.

Once, Anna said to me, "What would it have been like if a
woman you respected and admired told you, 'You know what
I like to do when I have my period? Put my feet up, make my
favorite cup of tea, and use a cozy blanket. Read a good book.
Honor my body'?"

I snorted. I hadn't heard people talk about their periods
that way.

✦

In her book *The Collected Schizophrenias*, Esmé Weijun Wang
writes: "Some people dislike diagnoses, disagreeably calling
them boxes and labels, but I've always found comfort in preex-
isting conditions; I like to know I'm not pioneering an inexpli-
cable experience."

Now that I had a name for what I was feeling, I was certain
I'd be able to control the outbursts with my mind. Sometimes
I'd even write myself letters while in non-PMDD weeks, to
read during an outburst, to remind myself it was only that.

In an interview, Erykah Badu said she put an alert on her
phone that would go off, reading: *Bitch, calm down, it's just
PMS.* I tried that, too, but I'd end up ignoring those alerts and
letters when the time actually came.

The night I found out about PMDD, I rested my computer

on the toilet while I took a bath, and watched YouTube videos of women talking about PMDD. There aren't hundreds, but there are some. I became so annoyed when a woman described all the same symptoms I had, only to say that what worked for her were calcium supplements and essential oils. I loved the sentiment, but it felt like such bullshit. Find me in the middle of a PMDD episode and hand me a bottle of essential oils and I promise you I will smash the bottle.

While researching, I came across something called the Gia Allemand Foundation for PMDD, which has since changed its name to the International Association for Premenstrual Disorders. Created in 2013, "The IAPMD aspires to create a world where people with PMDD and PME [premenstrual exacerbation] can survive and thrive." Even better, their website announced they'd be hosting a convention called Break the Cycle in May 2018 in Boca Raton, Florida. If you participated in some way, hosted a workshop or were a guest speaker, then the conference was free, save for the hotel.

I submitted a proposal to teach a writing workshop where I'd discuss "creative ways to work through PMDD." I was elated the conference existed. Maybe I had found my people. On our shared google calendar, Tony wrote CHLOE PMDD EXTRAVAGANZA to block out the week in May.

PART THREE

NUCLEAR FAMILY

"Here comes the nuclear family," my dad liked to say when the three of us walked into his music shop.

"Your dad posted a photo of us on Facebook," Tony would say occasionally.

"Which photo? What'd he say?"

"Something about having brunch with the nuclear family."

Curious, I thought. We weren't even close to being a nuclear family, if the definition of a nuclear family is a husband and wife who live with their child/children in one household.

"Here comes the nuclear family," he said from the counter, stringing a guitar or ringing up a customer for their Autoharp.

"The nuclear family's back together again?" he'd ask, if he hadn't seen us in a couple weeks, if we'd been out of town, or if Sadie hadn't been with us for a few days.

But did a nuclear family have a kid only two nights a week? Did a nuclear family have a not-quite stepparent? Didn't a nuclear family live together full-time? I still had my own apartment, four hundred and fifty-seven steps away.

"Here comes the blended family" would have been more accurate, but I suppose it doesn't have the same ring to it.

In the nuclear family my dad spoke of, every member had been through a divorce. Sadie and I were daughters of divorces, and Tony had been a firsthand participant.

Sadie had been part of a nuclear family until she was three. I'd been part of a nuclear family in my childhood, as well: a husband and wife, a boy and a girl.

My mom was an early childhood teacher and says the breaking up of the nuclear family was devastating to her. Divorce was uncommon then, and on paper she liked how the family looked: a carpenter, a teacher, two little kids two and a half years apart. Two of her sisters—she's sandwiched between them—had the same family structure, and they'd all met their husbands in high school. She broke the mold. I admire it, as it couldn't have been easy. Divorce: it can be the ultimate self-care.

The same year my dad moved out, my brother left for a boarding school, so we went from four people in our house to two: my mom and me.

Now, twenty years later, off the top of my head I can count an entire hand of Sadie's closest friends with divorced parents. It has become more uncommon for me to hear that someone's parents *are* still together. The family we hang out with most frequently consists of two gay men, one the adoptive father and the other the stepdad of a nine-year-old. When you ask the kid something about her dad, she often answers, "Which one?"

In an article for *The Atlantic*, David Brooks argues that the nuclear family is a mistake and a historical anomaly: "We take it as the norm, even though this wasn't the way most humans lived during the tens of thousands of years before 1950, and it isn't the way most humans have lived during the 55 years since 1965 . . . We think of kin as those biologically related to us. But throughout most of human history, kinship was something you could create."

Did my dad say it as a joke? Were we being mocked? Or was he mocking the stupidity of society? It also made a strange kind of sense; my dad was calling us what we looked like, instead of what we were. It was true that when we were in public, we could pass for a nuclear family.

The more I think about my dad and his name for us, the more I simply find my dad hilarious.

✦

The first time Tony called me "honey," I didn't know who he was speaking to. He had forgotten to fill the car with gas, which I was borrowing. "Sorry about that, honey," he said.

I was silent, frozen. Was he talking to Sadie? After some rumination I realized he was speaking to me. I'd never had a man or woman aside from my mother call me honey. I'd never heard my parents call each other honey. I simply didn't date people who called me honey.

✦

To say something happened overnight seems like a cliché, but Sadie and Tony started sleeping over, and overnight—literally—there were three toothbrushes in my yellow narcissus flower mug in the bathroom, after years of holding one.

A man held the door open for us at a restaurant where we were laughing about something. "I had to hold the door for you," he said, looking at me. "Because you look like such a happy family."

"Is that your daughter?" strangers on the street asked me, and when we were all ordering at a restaurant, the waiters directed questions to me about how Sadie wanted her food prepared, not looking at her dad.

Another time the three of us were sitting outside at a coffee shop, being loud and laughing, and a woman walked by and said we shouldn't be having so much fun.

A nuclear family was never in my list of dreams and goals, possibly a result of not just the divorce but also my generation.

To pass as a nuclear family is a privilege in some ways, just as passing as straight can be. On the other hand, passing for something other than you are also means you are not being seen, and not being seen can often hurt.

✦

One funny thing about Tony being from Wisconsin is that I did my fifth grade "choose a state" project on Wisconsin, solely for the reason that cheese was (and is) my favorite food. When I was twenty-one, I took a memoir writing class at Gotham Writers Workshop, and one of our assignments was to make a list of three things we were experts in. I can only remember one out of three—cheese. I suppose I thought I was an expert in things I loved. After class I left my notebook lying around our messy Brooklyn apartment and when Noelle saw my list, she laughed heartily and, not unkindly, said: "You're a *cheese* expert, dude?"

The June after meeting, we flew to Madison, Wisconsin, in the state of cheese, to visit (and for me to meet) Tony's parents. As I was retrieving Sadie's fidget spinner from the car, the word "hon" slipped out of my mouth. Sadie didn't freeze up exactly, but she didn't respond, either.

During our visit I was exposed to cheese curds for the first time (so I suppose I wasn't really a cheese expert, after all). I wasn't eating dairy for fear it caused my acne. It is wildly popular these days for people to say the hormones in dairy make you break out. In my experience, now eating a ton of cheese and having the clearest skin of my life, I think the whole dairy thing is a little too easy.

One afternoon, sitting on the patio having a Campari soda, Sadie crawled into my lap and asked, "Have you ever been married?"

"Nope," I said.

"If Dad got married again, I'd probably be the flower girl."

"Probably," I said.

✦

A week before we flew back home, Tony's mom told me that Sadie had told her, "Chloe's really nice. I'm not sure when she started calling me hon."

I knew what she meant. I wasn't sure when Tony started calling me honey either. Life felt like it was moving at triple the pace that it ever had before.

Driving through Madison one night, Tony had said, "I am excited about all aspects of life with you."

"Even the PMDD aspect?"

"Yep."

When we were walking through security, a TSA officer split us up, and told Tony to go through one door and Sadie and me to go through another.

"Mama and baby go that way, please," he said, getting both of our identities wrong. Sadie was a seven-year-old child who had to hold her own boarding pass. Sadie and I made eye contact; she put her hand over her mouth and giggled silently. We weren't mama and baby, we were something else, and that was our little secret.

We sat at our gate at the airport. Tony wanted to use the

bathroom and get a coffee. Sadie settled in next to me with her book. We both sipped jade cloud tea. "It's so much easier with three people," she said. "When it's just me and Dad I have to go everywhere with him—if he has to go to the bathroom, I have to go, and if he wants a coffee, I have to go. Now I get to stay here and have tea and read."

✦

My life became two extremes. First, being with Tony and Sadie: the chaos of flung bathing suits, the sound of feet pattering down the hall, the bursting open of our bedroom door at 6:00 a.m. Apple cinnamon oatmeal every morning; with milk, she'd remind me, not water. Macaroni and cheese was always about to be made, about to be eaten, or there were leftover pots of it on the stove.

Then: silence. Once they were gone, I'd be alone making the bed, doing the dishes, watering the plants, aimlessly pacing my apartment. My friend JD, who is engaged to a man with a daughter Sadie's age, told me it's like being ghosted, but by your boyfriend's kid. Sometimes Sadie would forget her Harry Potter scrunchie in my bathroom, and I'd use it to put up my hair at night when I washed my face.

It was almost like being single again, but it wasn't. Because they always came back.

WEREWOLF WEEK

r/PMDD
Now We Can All Feel Crazy Together! Arooooo
23.2K members
Created March 6, 2012

I wanna burn my house down and make little animals out of clay.

How bad is this supposed to get? I just tore the shower rod out of the wall.

I'm fucking stuck in this cycle: scream, cry, apologize, fuck, scream, cry, apologize, fuck.

This is not life—this is torture.

Last month I raged out and slammed the fridge door as hard as I could. Over and over and over again. I broke all the plastic door shelving and glass bottles shattered all over the floor.

I'm in Werewolf mode right now and I want to go to Sedona and see the foliage. I want to go alone.

It feels like my boobs are trying to suffocate me, my vagina is falling out, my back is stabbing me, and if that doesn't take me out, then I'll surely die from dehydration due to pre-period shits, coupled with the occasional vomit . . . also I'm pretty sure everyone I love hates me, and that I should run away.

I feel like the hulk going through an exorcism.

How the fuck am I only on Day 26 or maybe Day 27 holy fucking shit it feels like I'm on Day 32 This Is Fucking Maddening Holy Fucking Shit Sensory Nightmare Fuck Agh

I can't cope.

PMDD is ruining my life.

Need help coping with my desire to strangle everyone.

I am a 27 year old single woman with PMDD and ADHD. I have ruined every relationship I've ever been in due to my outbursts, even though when I am my sane self I am emotionally intelligent, kind, and a supportive partner (it usually feels one sided because my partners can't or don't know how to support me with my problems, and I've become reclusive and mostly given up on letting people in). I would like to create supportive relationships and friendships in my life that are not impacted by this illness, so I am considering getting my ovaries removed.

I feel so guilty for having PMDD and feeling like someone else controls my thoughts and emotions for days. I blow things up with my boyfriend and push him away but then that PMDD amnesia hits afterwards and I'm like, "Why are you upset?"

Don't you love it when you get the sudden urge to kill everyone?

A few questions for those of you that microdose psilocybin for PMDD: Do you microdose consistently through the month or only when you feel symptoms? When do you usually feel relief?

Monster has been the word I've been clicking with the last few days.

Luckily, my significant other is typically pretty understanding when it's PMDD time, and I think that makes a difference. We have a system where I put a red object on my desk when I'm having a particularly bad day, so he knows I'm struggling. Sometimes, when I don't even realize I'm in a bad mood, he'll say, "How many reds are you experiencing today." Lol! (Since he knows what PMDD is, he often notices my symptoms even before I do.)

I would have the whole reproductive shebang ripped out if I could. My hormones make me hate myself so much.

My mom doesn't believe me.

So, I no longer drink caffeine because during my PMDD I got into a fight at a dog park.

Do you ever just??? FFFEEELLL the PMDD enter your body???

Spilled a Dr Pepper and not only did I cry, but I threw the cloth napkin it spilt on across the room and screamed. I wanted to hit something else, but I didn't.

How do you decipher what's real and what's not during were-wolf week?

During werewolf week I have an aversion to men. This is probably made worse by the fact that I work with all men, but I seriously want them all to just piss off until I'm feeling more like a normal human. I get into a room with all women, and I swear I can literally feel my blood pressure drop.

You have to be committed to looking through the lies that the "werewolf" tells you.

Werewolf is telling me to dump my boyfriend and give up on AP tests.

PMDD made me lose my shit over banana bread today.

Improving but lonely: Am I the only werewolf in the world? Also, I'm SO ALONE in this. I have never met a person with PMDD in real life. I don't even know any women who will admit to having PMS problems at all.

Birth control has controlled Werewolf Week for almost 4 years, so I'm stunned by this relapse.

Just survived the worst werewolf week I've had in a long time!!!

Anybody get tingling in their limbs during werewolf week?

Starting Prozac, will I become a person again?

I hate it cause when my daughter sees it makes me feel like complete shit. I always talk with her after and explain, she's so sweet! I feel like a horrible person and parent when I let this take me over.

There are men on this sub who browse here for their partners, who are lovely, caring, empathetic individuals. A lot of them browse here for advice to best support their partners. If what they see is an echo chamber of women hating men, or insinuating that they should tolerate all behavior, or that they can't say or voice concerns, then it will dissuade them from moving forward helping their partner with PMDD. Our partners need to be empathetic, yes, but they are not punching bags, and they cannot be expected to tolerate all behavior, and should be allowed to speak up if they are concerned.

I finally found you all. I could cry.

My daily supplement cocktail to help with werewolf week(s). What meds / supplements help you calm the pmdd monster?

1. Calcium / Magnesium / Zinc
2. 5-HTP
3. Rhodiola Rosea
4. Probiotics + Chaga Mushroom
5. Ashwagandha
6. GABA
7. Dopa Mucuna
8. Fo-Ti Root
9. Vitex
10. L-Tyrosine

11. L-Theanine

12. w33d

I make sure I'm hitting all magnesium, potassium, zinc, calcium, sodium, vit d goals daily. Through food/sun exposure. I am also extremely intentional about eliminating/recognizing stressors in my life. They heighten all symptoms.

Heal your inner child and all that stuff, Google it.

THINGS LIKE BANANA BREAD PMDD MADE ME LOSE MY SHIT OVER

Chicken lo mein

The "right" way to make nachos

If we were making soup or not

That I looked bad in a photo where I'm holding a Vitaminwater

THE MAGIC BULLET

I'd quit caffeine. I went to yoga regularly and occasionally Quaker meetings, which were held a couple of blocks from my apartment. I finally did the (goddamn) Whole30. I'd read books like *Dark Nights of the Soul*. Anna, my therapist, had become trained in EMDR and we did a few sessions. She invited me to a group therapy with other women-identifying people, which I attended monthly. The somatic therapy I'd been doing regularly with her was enlightening and challenging. I saw progress. Everything helped, but not enough. My therapist agreed; she'd seen my lifestyle changes and how hard I was working, and though she doesn't prescribe medication, she agreed I didn't need to keep suffering for something I possibly inherited.

I relate to a friend who had a breast reduction—she told me she just woke up one morning and made the decision. Enough of the suffering and muscling through, and enough of the idea in the back of her head that she'd do it "someday." Someday was now.

The day I finally procured Prozac, I had therapy first. I began to cry, discussing the previous night of PMDD. Whenever I begin crying during therapy, though, I make myself stop. I don't want to waste my time and money crying instead of talking—I can cry for free any day of the week.

Back at my cold apartment (cold because my landlady had written in the lease that in the winter the heat would stay at sixty-five degrees. I'm more of a seventy-three-degree person in the winter, but it wasn't up to me. Tony thinks it was because she was going through menopause, so she was running hot to my cold), I called one of my friends who has been taking Prozac for years. While we chatted I put on two sweaters, mittens, a scarf, a hat, and sunglasses. I walked to my doctor's office ten minutes away, up the hill at the hospital. Everyone in the waiting room had gray hair and wedding rings on their hands. People were coughing.

I had bitched about my previous doctor's lack of knowledge of PMDD to my therapist, who had then recommended her own doctor. She told me the doctor wasn't for everyone—she was a little snide and told you exactly what to do and was more on the naturopathic side of medicine. I'd decided to switch over to her.

✦

Whenever I think about when my PMDD began developing, I return to my memories of the August before I met Tony. I was thirty; the summer was hormonally horrific. I was cat-sitting down in Brooklyn for the month. The feta went bad in the fridge. I skimmed on my phone how to make hard-boiled eggs and a year later realized I'd read it wrong—you do not boil the eggs for twenty minutes; you let them *sit* for twenty minutes. So the whole summer my eggs were overcooked and smelly.

When I got back upstate, I'd driven to my mom's house. My mother was sitting in the grass. She looked small, like a child. I leaned against my car, too angry to sit, every cell in my body flaring. Explosive. I told my mom something about wanting to try antidepressants. She argued that I didn't have depression, just anxiety. *Just.*

"Untreated anxiety turns into depression!" I screamed. "How can you say I don't have depression? You're medicated, people in your family are medicated!"

"*My* family has depression," she said, emphasizing "my," referring to her seven siblings and parents.

"*I come from your family!*" I wonder how this sounded. I'm tempted to say I bellowed.

Even though I hadn't even made it into the house yet, I peeled out of the driveway. I haven't used that phrase—"peeled out"—since high school, but that is what happened.

Later my mom emailed an apology of sorts, said she needed to work on her expectations, that she was excited to see me and to go to the book fair, that she had made chicken salad. This detail always stuck with me: *I had made chicken salad. I had made chicken salad for us.*

Except instead of writing out the full word chicken, she wrote *chix.*

We can be in a monumental fight and still use shorthand with each other.

✦

The doctor's assistant, Sam, brought me in. She asked where I was in my cycle. She asked what my symptoms were. I told her about the rage, the panic, the tears out of nowhere. I knew she knew something about all this. I could see it in her eyes.

I'd still been conflicted about going on medication. I *was* conditioned to think antidepressants were for weaker people. On some level I probably felt superior for not being on antidepressants. Even though my friends were on them. Even though writers I admired were on them. Even though my family members were on them.

The kicker for me was in December 2017 when I read the novel *Motherhood* by Sheila Heti. I'd been sent an early copy of the novel and stayed up until 3:00 a.m. devouring it. The book is about the fluctuations of the narrator's desire to have a baby depending on her changing hormones during her cycle. Eventually, the narrator realizes that there are women out there experiencing what she's experiencing, and she goes on medication. You can imagine my disbelief, my excitement. I was moved to email Sheila, whom I'd been in touch with occasionally in the past, a letter of admiration and gratitude for her book.

She told me she'd read *Listening to Prozac* by Peter D. Kramer and that it shifted her thinking of medication; she didn't see it as a failure anymore.

Sheila recommended I try taking maca in water or smoothies every day. She said it was the only potion-like thing that actually helped her PMS, and sent me a picture. I told her sweet potatoes work for me, or at least I think they do.

She said: "Prozac is the 'cleanest' of the serotonin-boosting drugs. Go with the very lowest dose if you decide on it—10 mg."

She said: "It's like taking a little bit of sunshine."

Getting the blessing from her, a woman who had written a book *while* taking Prozac—debunking the myth that if you go on meds your creativity will disappear—settled my conflict. She hadn't met me with shame, but with strength. The kindness and kinship she showed me that winter were memorable.

✦

My new doctor entered the room, and I asked her if anyone had ever told her she looked like Rachel Griffiths, who

plays Brenda Chenowith in *Six Feet Under*. She had no idea
who I was talking about, but I thought I loosened her up.
She wrote down a list of foods I should cut out of my diet. I
lied and told her I'd already cut out caffeine and dairy, even
though earlier that day I'd had two cafés au lait at the coffee
shop.

> Dairy
>
> Caffeine
>
> Sugar
>
> Alcohol
>
> Gluten
>
> Wheat

"It is difficult to live on organic meat and greens when you're
broke," I told her. I either said "poor" or "broke." Clearly, my
privilege and race affect my ability to be able to walk into a
doctor's office and demand to be listened to. I still tend to get
dramatic in doctor's offices, because I am speaking from a defensive place, already thinking the doctor does not believe me.

Dr. Wallace seemed different, though.

She asked if the yogurt I eat was sweetened or unsweet-
ened. She asked if I chewed gum, and what brand. Did I sleep
with my mouth open or closed? Did I buy vitamins off Am-
azon? Because I definitely should not. I also should not be
using the plastic water bottle I was carrying. (I recycled it

when I got home.) She told me about a special kind of tape you can buy to tape your mouth shut at night, because if you sleep with your mouth even slightly open, you lose the good bacteria in your mouth. For breakfast, she told me, she had a small piece of organic steak, and eggs and greens. It sounded delicious.

Dr. Wallace believed me about the PMDD. The seriousness of it. "There's a kid involved," I told her, choking up, and I was surprised when she asked how old. She was listening.

She said she would let me try generic Prozac but thought I would see more relief with diet. Every time I countered what she said, she countered me back. She didn't back down and neither did I. But we respected each other by the end of the appointment.

Asking for a prescription reminded me of when you try to get out of a ticket from a cop. Like you're kind of making yourself cry in a fake way but you're also actually crying. Women are infamously ignored, degraded, and condescended to in doctor's offices, so even when someone believes you, it is hard to believe they believe you.

I took the blood work request to the basement. The woman behind the counter looked at my papers and said, "You're not going to have any blood left after this!"

In the parking lot, I read the piece of paper Dr. Wallace had given me.

PMDD (Premenstrual Dysphoric Disorder)
Cystic acne

I sat and stared at it for a while. I took a photograph of it because it felt like a true selfie. I considered sending it to people but kept it to myself.

✦

The comedian Jacqueline Novak has said on her podcast that having to haul your depressed ass to the drugstore to pick up meds is an indignity. I agree. Clearly if you're picking up meds for the first time, something is wrong. They should be delivered to your doorstep in a basket with some magazines and bubble bath, kind of like how they deliver meals in a basket to your door at MacDowell, the artist's residency in New Hampshire. Or so I've heard.

In the past, I bonded with romantic partners by asking, "Have you ever been on medication?"

"Nope. Just been self-medicating for a long time," they'd respond. (I had a type.)

"Me, too!" I'd say, glad that we were both on the crazy spectrum, but not the kind of *basic* crazy who needed mainstream meds. Looking back, I cringe at my naivete, my judgement.

When I finally got home, I was depleted from talking

about my mental health all day. When I was little my mom taught me the term "mental health day." She'd let me take off school and go into work with her where she taught preschool. We'd always stop at a corner store for snacks. Now, mental health day seemed to take on a new meaning.

My mom sent me a voice memo about something unrelated, and I felt emboldened to write back and ask her which antidepressants she'd tried in her life, which I'd never asked her before.

Her message back sounded frustrated and annoyed. "I don't know Chlo, there isn't a magic bullet."

As if I'm naive enough to think there's a magic bullet! I don't think this is fair—to be on antidepressants and also tell me I don't need them. It was so clear what was going on: she didn't want to have a daughter on Prozac. A daughter with a book out, with a boyfriend, with her own apartment, sure. But not a daughter on Prozac.

At the same time, maybe I *was* naive enough to think there was a magic bullet. That was why I continued to read Reddit, order supplements, try new ways of eating.

✦

In the year 2000, the FDA approved Prozac as the only antidepressant suitable for treating PMDD. It was rebranded as the more feminine-sounding Sarafem but made with identical ingredients to Prozac, just colored pink, because god forbid a woman take a pill that isn't pink. When people with PMDD were given Prozac, 80 percent felt better. Some only take it beginning the day they ovulate until the onset of menstruation. When serotonin is blocked in the brain, the result is strikingly similar to PMDD symptoms, so it makes sense that an SSRI would treat both issues.

A commercial: As a woman struggles to get a cart outside the grocery store, a voice-over begins. "Think about the week before your period. Do you feel irritably? Tension? Tiredness? Think it's PMS? Think again. It could be PMDD."

A woman runs down the stairs while a voice says: "It's back. The week before your period." The woman searches in her bag frantically, then looks up, annoyed, saying, "Did you take my keys?" presumably to her husband. She finds her keys in her coat pocket and heads out the door.

Is that a depiction of PMDD? Or of a person just looking for her keys?

Eli Lilly, the manufacturer of Prozac, pulled the ads after the Food and Drug Administration castigated the company for marketing the drug too aggressively. The agency said the commercial pitched the medicine to women who had normal PMS and thereby trivialized the seriousness of premenstrual dysphoric disorder.

◆

I swallowed my first Prozac at night even though the directions say to take it in the morning because I can't follow directions. Then I climbed into my bathtub for warmth. Except the hot water in my apartment runs out quickly, so I boiled water in the teakettle on the stove and brought it into the bathroom with me to periodically pour into the bathtub. How's that for a hack?

THE OPPOSITE OF LIGHT
(A PROZAC DIARY)

The kitchen—it happened in the kitchen. I was drinking Sweet Tangerine Positive Energy tea—because I need all the help I can get—and I noticed, though it was a six-degree day and snowing, that I was having positive thoughts about spring.

How beautiful spring is. How cool that spring comes after winter! What an amazing cycle!

Normally I stand in front of my space heater and think about how cold it is, how much I detest the cold, how much harder the cold makes simple tasks, how terrible winter is, how difficult life is, *what's the point of anything?*

Music is sounding better than usual, has more depth. I noticed myself loudly singing along.

One woman's Zoloft is another woman's Prozac.

Dr. Diana L. Dell in *The PMDD Phenomenon*:

> When a person first takes an SSRI, serotonin
> levels begin to increase over twelve to twenty-
> four hours. It is not enough to treat major
> depressives, but it is enough to treat women
> with PMS or PMDD. Clinically, women say
> by the time they seek medical treatment for
> their severe symptoms, many women are so
> discouraged by the lack of improvement af-
> ter trying self-help treatments that they don't
> expect the medication to work either. When
> their next menstrual cycle comes with none
> of their usual premenstrual symptoms, they
> report being shocked and delighted.

Just as people only read political articles that reiterate their
opinion, I'm reading only Prozac success stories.

My digestion is improving, which also makes me happier.
Maybe that's been the problem. Maybe not shitting every day
was making me a moody bitch. In fact, I have to poop right
now! I even found myself googling "I love Prozac" on the toilet.

Later I caught myself skipping in the kitchen. Shocked and
delighted. Then dancing in the living room. My acne is flaring

because it is werewolf week but it isn't upsetting me as much as usual. I find myself saying things to myself like, "Oh well! It will pass!" Earlier my car wouldn't start even with a jump, and Tony texted me, "Oh no! That sucks!" and I was like, "It's okay! It will probably start when the weather warms tomorrow."

Is this how Tony always feels? Not *always*, but is it his baseline? How frustrating I must be for him if this is his natural state.

I wonder if the voice of this book is changing now that I'm on Prozac.

I feel warm today. I am drinking my maca and texting with about four girlfriends and my love for them is vast. I went to hot yoga yesterday and it felt wonderful. If I could just give Tony a month where I don't have an outburst, it would be the best birthday gift I could give him. Though just in case, I also got us tickets to see a comedy show in March.

It's funny when you turn into the thing that you are fascinated by and also fear. The woman whose car is always fucked up. The woman who takes supplements. The woman who goes on antidepressants.

It makes sense I'd end up on Prozac. Since I was a teenager, I always found pills to be remarkable. Sure, I liked snorting stuff,

too, because it was exciting and dirty and wrong and glamorous, but swallowing a pill that you know will kick in a bit later
and give you a "sense of well-being" is pretty much the best
feeling in the world. It is so easy to do. It takes less than a second and you can do it while talking to someone and they don't
even notice. You don't even have to go to the bathroom to do
it. I loved how the letters looked on Vicodin and Valium, the
friendly curve of the V, the soft blue of Valium, the pure white
of Vicodin. It is my good fortune that I've never broken a bone
or had back problems because if I got a prescription for that
stuff, I would go nowhere fast.

I've gotten really into texting the rainbow emoji, an emoji I'd
never texted before. Rainbows, suns, and hearts. Mostly
rainbows.

From *Prozac Diary* by Lauren Slater: "I fell in love one day,
only it was not with a person; it was with my pill. Stark naked
and delightfully drugged, I sat in that bath of bubbles. I bit into
an apple, and I enjoyed the gesture . . . Prozac brought me to
pumpkin muffins, yellowfin tuna, and plum sauce."

And then, a miracle: I got my period the day before Tony's
birthday, eight days into my Prozac experiment, with barely
a glimmer of regular PMS. I was sitting on my therapist's
couch—not crying!—when I began to feel some cramps. "I am

glad," she said, as I pulled my boots on to leave, "that you are feeling more buoyant."

"You," Tony said, across from me at dinner, "are doing really well. Your mood is so even; it's wild." I was ecstatic for days after. I'd gotten through my period without collateral damage. It is so . . . relaxing.

On his birthday we had a lovely morning of sleeping in and coffee, an afternoon walk through the snow at a nature conservatory, and a silly and romantic dinner out. Sure, I took a couple of Advil for cramps and had some minor irritability—but it was so minor that I'm not even sure I had any. And after living through what feels like a nightmare on earth, I welcome any regular irritability with open-as-fuck arms.

✦

January feels like it's been going on forever. The most exciting thing that has happened—aside from the Prozac—is that I received an email saying my proposal was accepted for the PMDD convention. Now I'll have to figure out how the hell to teach a PMDD writing workshop.

Tony laughed yesterday because I wanted to keep tracking the yellow couch we ordered.

"I love tracking things," I said.

"Yup, you track your period, you track your packages," he said.

From *Prozac Nation* by Elizabeth Wurtzel: "I can't help feeling that anything that works so effectively, that's so transformative, has got to be hurting me at another end, maybe sometime further down the road."

It is *still* January. Tony's been out of town for over a week and we haven't had conflict over text. It feels incredible. Is this sustainable?

✦

Nope. It was a little too good to be true. It's February; rabbit rabbit. I spent the morning reading Instagram posts under the hashtag #periodssuck and started following someone named @Pmddsufferer. I've also found: @Pmddmama, @pmdd.india, @pmddzone, @pmdd.is.a.thing, @pmddloveandlight, @pmddrainbow, @pmddpositive, @pmdd_queen, @pmddsupport, @lifewithpmdd, @pmddisnotincontrol, @pmddadvocacy, @pmdd.survivor, @pmdd.memes, @mypmddhell, @pmddawareness, @pmddpoetry, @pmddwitch, @pmddhaven, @pmdddiaries, @pmdddaze, @pmdd.nederland, @pmddhealthcoach, @pmddhealthtips, @pmddcanada,

@pmdd_endo_warrior, @pmdd_with_a_migraine, @pmd-
dwhispers, @pmddwomen, @pmddguru, @pmdd_recov-
ernaturally, @surviving.pmdd, @living_with_pmdd, and
@myuterushatesme.

"Well, folks, it looks like we arrived at our PMDD destination a little early. Don't hit your head getting off the platform,"
Tony said, sending me Bitmoji of him getting hit with bombs.

"Fuck off."

"Omg. I'm joking."

"It's funny but still."

"I'm trying to be nice."

"That's your way of being nice?"

My therapist says that each time we think we've finished one
piece of work, another piece of work presents itself. There is
always another layer, and we are never done.

On February 14 we drove to Lisbon, Connecticut, to purchase
a bed Tony found on Facebook Marketplace. We were arguing
about something we'd already argued about a few times. Except

this time, it was Valentine's Day and our bed frame was pushing up into the front of the car, dividing our faces, a piece of wood between us so we couldn't see each other's eyes. We started laughing and it was all unexpectedly romantic. That night we got couple's massages and we couldn't stop giggling at something stupid.

Tony left for work in Aspen and after he landed had to take a three-hour car ride. He was driving through the mountains while we text-fought and he said, "This is the same energy you gave me the last time I drove through the mountains," which, in retrospect, is sort of funny. What is my problem when he drives through the mountains? Is it because he is experiencing something without me? When we are both in Hudson, we are together every day and eat dinner together almost every night. Probably six out of seven nights a week, if not seven. So I guess I was just adjusting to knowing I would now be alone for three weeks. He'd always come back from traveling with pockets full of receipts and Stroopwaffles. In some ways I liked when he went to Colorado because he'd bring me back THC salve for my cramps.

"Airplane Mode," he texted me, which was our new tool when we were fighting. He'd then go into Airplane Mode and wait a few hours until whatever I was going through had passed. I'd use Airplane Mode, too, when I needed space or to ground.

Sadie and I were collaging a ukulele with designs and pictures cut out from magazines, using Mod Podge glue. Each time she had to use the Mod Podge, she'd walk around the table to get it. "I'm going to move this closer to you," I said, putting the glue in front of her. "It'll make your life easier."

Outside it snowed. We had a quiet moment.

"It's funny how people say that," she said. "Like, it will make my entire *life* easier?"

She had a really good point, and I thought it was a really deep thing for a seven-year-old to contemplate.

As you get older, you're constantly making choices that can make your life 5 percent harder or easier. Over time, you realize you cannot control most of your life, so you do the things you can control, like moving the glue closer.

Sadie gave me a stack of papers to look over out of her Friday Folder for school. Later that night, drinking my rose tea (which on the box claims to be "magical" and "stress-relieving"), I saw her bonus word was "cramping." She got it right, giving her another three points.

She fell asleep in bed with me last night since Tony was gone. All night I dreamed of blood running down my leg. I was also dreaming of flying on an airplane, being at the airport, of friends, but in the back of my mind was worry I was bleeding down my left leg, bleeding on the sheets, bleeding through my underwear. I went to the bathroom three times to check, and I was imagining it every time save for the small, circular blood-stain on my gray Victoria's Secret underwear.

Sadie recently asked me what my latest essay was about.

"Complicated things you go through as an adult. Problems you may have. Hormones, moods, stuff like that."

"Oh, so it's like the opposite of light."

Tony and I caught eyes.

"What do you mean, 'the opposite of light'?" I asked.

"Well, it's the opposite of what I write."

"What do you write?"

"Like, essays about autumn, for example."

THINGS THAT HELPED BUT ALSO WHO REALLY KNOWS SINCE TREATMENT ENDED UP BEING SUCH A LAYERED APPROACH?

Maca powder in smoothies and water

Pure Encapsulations iodine supplements

Sweet potatoes with cinnamon and ghee for breakfast

Sliced turkey

10mg of Prozac

Chugging raspberry tea

Airplane Mode

Long walks every day and/or especially leading up to period

Floradix iron supplements

Jenny Hval's albums *Blood Bitch* and *Apocalypse, girl*

Eating a rotisserie chicken in the car when the blood begins to come on

C U Later Dysphoria tincture from 69herbs

There were a few times Tony and I would take an edible and somehow end up reading the PMS Reddit group aloud and be in hysterics. We'd search #PMS on TikTok and cry laughing. We felt seen.

Stratos CBD and THC hybrid tablets (but weed often frightened me, as I was concerned it would bring on more paranoia)

Vitamin D Liquid by Thorne

CALM Magnesium

THINGS THAT DIDN'T HELP

Some women on the PMDD subgroup of Reddit say they wear a piece of jewelry, like a bracelet or a ring that they normally never wear, or buy it specifically for this reason. Then you wear the bracelet or ring to remind you it isn't your real anxiety, it's your PMDD anxiety.

Vape pens seemed to help lots of people but I was concerned they'd heighten my paranoia.

Writing myself letters during non-PMDD to read during PMDD

Drinking entire pots of French press coffee first thing, phone in hand

Cold brew all day, phone in hand

PMS Ease Synergy Blend essential oils by Edens Garden

Nature Bright Sun Touch Plus light and negative ionizer

DIM supplements

For the lock screen on my phone, I put a photo of Sadie I'd taken in Wisconsin, where she is standing in front of a mural that reads COMPASSION and smiling sweetly. I thought it would help me find compassion for those rageful moments. It didn't help.

Chasteberry supplements

PART FOUR

BANANA SPLITS

"I don't want to go through another divorce," I'd tell Tony from time to time.

"Can you say that same statement as a positive?"

"I want to stay together," I'd sigh reluctantly.

"That's better."

When waiters would refer to Tony as my "husband" I'd make a show of acting disgusted, as if the word made me want to throw up. Another time, we were at a bank and the teller talking to Tony referred to me as "your wife" and I bristled, rolled my eyes. Tony didn't flinch.

I was a walking contradiction, though. One afternoon at the library a few blocks from my apartment, I checked out the book *Passionate Marriage* by David Schnarch. Some nights I read it in bed with Sadie and Tony during what we called "reading parties." I appreciated how neither of them said anything or seemed to notice the book and its title.

✦

Banana Splits is a school-based children's group program established in 1978 by social worker Liz McGonagle for students who have experienced parental divorce or death. In elementary school, I remember an aide or guidance counselor would periodically pop into the classroom and announce it was time for Banana Splits. I liked the name, the double meaning, even then. It seemed special, just as braces and glasses were special. Certain kids would screech their chairs back, grab their backpacks, and leave.

In adulthood I heard from a friend that her schools had a similar program for children of divorce—except it was called Broken Rainbows.

In the past few years when I learned divorce is the second most traumatic event after death and before moving, I was shocked. had no clue. No one told me. I'd downplayed it my whole life. Now, Sadie was a reflection of the back and forth—living out of your backpack, never fully relaxing on transition days because you know you'll soon have to pack up, your mom at the bottom of the stairs at your dad's apartment, your dad waiting in the car at your mom's house.

My parents weren't split up when I was in elementary school, though. By the time they were, I was in ninth grade and I don't think Banana Splits was offered anymore. Plus, if they had offered it when I was a teenager, you can be sure I wouldn't have gone. I was the queen of blowing things off then, of not showing up, skipping.

When my parents separated (they didn't divorce until about thirteen years later), there was nothing interesting about it to my fourteen-year-old brain. There was nothing interesting about divorce to me, just as there was nothing interesting about my period. I was not searching, exploring, or mining these events. I was not digging; I was only surviving.

At times I envy the new generation—how normalized therapy and divorce are, even for kids, especially for kids in blended families, how there isn't drama or an air of taboo around it. Back in 2000, when my parents separated, I didn't have a mirror for what my family looked like. I'd never even seen *Kramer vs. Kramer*. *The Squid and the Whale* wasn't released until 2005, after I'd already graduated high school. TGFJBB. (Thank god for Judy Blume books.) My favorites were *It's Not the End of the World* and *Just as Long as We're Together*.

The lack wasn't loving parents—I won the lottery in that department—the lack was a community. Resources. The lack was having a language for it. The lack was having vocabulary.

It's a funny thing, shame. You don't always know you're feeling it until it's too late.

Sometimes I look at Sadie and see the enormous number of role models and mentors she has: her four parents, two grandmothers, guitar teacher, women on TV. Sadie is queen of watching media with a Strong Female Lead.

When I was fourteen, I went with my mom to the DMV. I spent a lot of time after school at appointments with my mom so she could change her legal last name from the last name we shared back to her maiden name.

"Never change your last name," I remember her saying, implying it was such a pain in the ass to change it back.

On December 19, 2017, I received the following email:

Did you forget?

Our records indicate that the following item(s) are overdue.
Please return them as soon as you can in order to minimize the fines which you may owe.

AUTHOR: Schnarch, David Morris,
Passionate marriage : love, sex, an
CALL NO: 616.891 Sch
BARCODE: 32390004603830
Adriance Adult DUE: 12-05-17
DATE CHECKED OUT: 11-14-17 04:11PM

But I didn't know where the book was, and I didn't want to give it back. I vaguely remembered keeping it in my car, under a bunch of garbage.

✦

Even now, I am hearing a judgmental voice saying, *Shut up.*
It was only a divorce! Millions of people have them. Kids survive
them. Don't get me wrong: Divorce is one of the most brilliant
concepts out there. It was good for me to see my mom know
herself well enough to know that the hardship of divorce was
better than staying in an unhappy marriage. That's one thing
I never related to in Judy Blume books, and Sadie has said
the same thing: the protagonist's motivation is always to get
their parents back together. I never wanted my parents back
together. I didn't mourn the nuclear family. Something I don't
have a name for was still lost, though. Even now, twenty-one
years later, I *still* lack the language.

◆

In "Growing up in the Divorced Family," Dr. Judith S. Wallerstein finds that the largest impact from divorce occurs during
the period in which the child of divorce is a young adult wanting a romantic relationship but afraid of failure.

Wallerstein coined the term "sleeper effect": "the phenomenon whereby individuals who previously showed positive
recovery following childhood parental divorce later exhibit ad-
justment difficulties in young adulthood stemming from the
earlier experience of parental divorce." She cites longitudinal
research that suggests that "as children of divorce enter adulthood, they may be more likely than the general population to

experience concerns about not being loved, have difficulties in relationship formation and maintenance, and have fears regarding betrayal and abandonment in romantic relationships."

The sleeper effect was definitely exacerbated for me by the way I smoked pot every day.

Dr. E. Mavis Hetherington disagrees. Her work attempts to dispel the notion that divorce is always negative. She has a chapter in her book *For Better or For Worse* called "Mostly Happy: Children of Divorce as Young Adults." Her theory is that Wallerstein exaggerates the effect of divorce on children, and that most children recover quickly. "Divorcing is a high-risk situation," Dr. Hetherington writes, "but the majority of divorced parents and their children are resilient and able to cope with the challenges in their postdivorce life."

I see both sides, and appreciate both perspectives. Both things can be true: divorce can be positive for the overall family, over time, but can also have negative repercussions on the kids, if kids don't have sufficient support.

My therapist once gave me the assignment of making a list of couples whom I knew who were happily married. It was tough and uncomfortable, the way it sounds when friends tell me their therapist has them say "I love you" every day in the mirror. I couldn't think of more than three couples in my life to put on the list. I included my therapist, because I knew that she was married with two kids—a true nuclear family.

One night in bed I came across this in "Growing up in the

Divorced Family": "One third of the men and women were openly pessimistic about marriage and divorce and sought to avoid both."

It was true. In my twenties and early thirties, my mantra was "I don't want to get married because I don't want to get divorced." To me, marriage was synonymous with divorce. Why is that surprising? What else did I know? Tony's parents have been together for fifty years, so he expected to stay together.

On a walk discussing this notion, Tony reminded me that he'd *also* been through divorce but still wasn't afraid of it. I imagine this is because *choosing* to get a divorce is a different experience than being pulled along for someone else's.

I remember an evening I was on my porch where I'd just moved in with Tony. I was having wine with a friend, and I explained that in my skewed view, moving in with someone, which I knew on paper was exciting to most people, was *the beginning of the end.*

She laughed in disbelief. Her parents were divorced, too. "That is so incredibly fucked up," she said. She continued: "I'm fucked up but that is *really* fucked up." We kept laughing.

✦

One summer I took Tony and Sadie to Gloucester, Massachusetts, where I'd gone with my aunts, mom, and cousins every year for over a decade, and we stayed for three nights.

Over dinner at Lobsta Land, Sadie told us she couldn't picture a life with her parents together. I told her *same*. She told us she was glad not to be around bickering. I told her *same*. She said she has a memory of when her dad came back to her mom's house and told them he'd found an apartment. I told her *same*.

In the article "Children After Divorce" in *The New York Times*, Dr. Wallerstein writes:

"Children of divorce have vivid memories about their parents' separation. The details are etched firmly in their minds, more so than those of any other experiences in their lives."

My mom says it was not the loss of the marriage (good marriages don't end) but the loss of the formation of family. She has told me that she'd become bleakest at 5:00 p.m., when most families are cooking, convening, conversing over dinner. Instead, she was alone in our cold house. She said sometimes she'd go to the library after work just to use their heat.

My mom and I both listened to an episode of *The KICK-ASS Stepmom Podcast* where two women my age, Jamie Scrimgeour and Laura Epstein, spoke about nearly identical experiences to mine. "We always fall back on saying: *kids are resilient, kids are resilient*. Can we stop with that for a second?" one of the women said.

My mom said it brought her to tears. "Divorce is so powerful and heartbreaking," she texted me after.

Then she texted, "Did I ever ask u if u were ok."

"I don't remember."

A theory: when I stopped numbing myself, which I had done from age fifteen to thirty in various and impressive ways, the uncomfortable parts of life, the stuff I'd never dealt with, the divorce I'd never looked at, came coursing through my veins. The paranoia, hypervigilance, and anxiety that I didn't have support for when I was a teenager releases now once a month when my hormones crash, and those feelings of emotional unsafety come out as rage. Often people go into anger because they are afraid of what's underneath. And often what's underneath is terror.

◆

Instagram alerts me that I have a new memory, and that I can review it. What does that mean, to review a memory?

Did you forget? the library asks again.

In the article by Wallerstein, I read: "We were stunned when, at the second series of visits, we found family after family still in crisis, their wounds wide open. Turmoil and distress had not noticeably subsided. Many adults were angry, and felt humiliated and rejected."

Humiliated and rejected? I used the same phrasing during an outburst with Tony (an outburst you can read about in an earlier chapter).

◆

My heart breaks for the resources my mom and I didn't have back in the early 2000s; it was like the blind leading the blind. Now, just type "divorce" into your podcast app for dozens of episodes and podcasts like *Moms Moving On, Divorce and Your Money, Surviving Divorce Podcast*. I so wonder what it is like to be a teenager and secretly listening to these. I wonder if I would have felt better about myself. My mom told me she had read *When Things Fall Apart* by Pema Chödrön. When I tell people my mom pitched a tent at Kripalu and brought Pema Chödrön with her, they tell me my mom is their hero.

Divorce doesn't explain everything, of course, yet I also want to honor its impact. I'm a fan of divorce: isn't it divorce that led me to my family? It doesn't only break families up; it brings other families together. Blended, nuclear, broken, chosen, step, bonus, tomato, tomato potato, potato.

Did you forget?

I did forget. And then I remembered.

On January 3, 2018, I received another email from the library:

> THIS REQUIRES YOUR IMMEDIATE
> ATTENTION
> This is a bill for the replacement cost(s) of the following item(s) which have not been returned

Passionate marriage : love, sex, and intimacy
in emotionally committed
REPLACEMENT Adriance Adult 3239000
4603830...........................$21.05
TOTAL$21.05

I figured a passionate marriage was worth $21.05, so I just
paid it off. That night, Tony had one of his sleeptalking bouts.
"Never lie to an artist," I heard him say.

A KNIFE IN THE ASS

r/PMDDpartners
A community for the partners of people who suffer from PMDD.
A place to ask for advice, or just to vent about your experience with
PMDD.
616 members
Created August 18, 2017

What a knife in the ass all this is.

The psychological warfare could do a partner's head in for sure.

It's an intensity and ferocity that comes on seemingly out of nowhere. I try to remember that it will pass though in the moment it is incredibly challenging and often infuriating. Meeting it with love and knowing how to kindly walk away and not engage have helped though can be difficult to remember and act upon in the moment.

The journey with PMDD has been one with its own ups and downs. It was most difficult before we knew what we were dealing with. I really just thought my wife hated me for 1-2 weeks every month, and thought she was going to break up with me. It wasn't until I noticed that these times were happening in a cyclical fashion that we started to make progress. After that, we started growing together.

It is unreal. Sometimes I think it's easier for her to let PMDD fuck everything up than try to rein it in.

How the fuck are 2 people supposed to live together when at any moment the sufferers brain gets hijacked without anyone knowing until you are already in a horrible fight . . . Then the PMDD's existence gets denied by the sufferer for a week. Then forgotten about till next week when you are at each other's throats again. Wtf kind of sick joke is this shit?

She will say she's sorry for acting "a little crazy" days later but she won't seek help or see the full extent of her raging. During counseling she just said she gets moody sometimes. She downplays the entire situation.

It hurts to endure the switch . . . I still love her though.

It's tough to remember the good times, especially during the dark days. Remember though, as tough as it is for us, it's even worse for our partners.

It goes against every fiber in my being to do this, but sometimes I wish I could record my wife when she's like this so I can show it to her when she's not. She simply does not remember.

We've been to multiple doctors. Half of them don't even know what PMDD is and seem skeptical when you explain it. Right now, they have her on Prozac, but it's not helping as far as living a normal life.

PMDD is a condition, it's not a curse and it doesn't need to define someone, or define your relationship. I know several women who manage to live fulfilling lives with it and keep their relationships intact.

Just can't handle this anymore. I've tried to be supportive for the last 8 years now, but I can't keep doing this. It's sapping my will to live.

Yesterday, I thought I would pick up a bottle of wine as a surprise for her. I'd taken a photo of her favorite bottle so I wouldn't forget it. I barely drink, and usually she buys wine for herself - but I thought it might be nice to share a bottle and have a relaxing evening.

We sit down, and she tells me that me buying her wine as a gift is triggering because her ex (who she endlessly compares everything to) used to give her alcohol to try and up his odds that they would have sex. I said that I was sorry that made her feel that way, and it was not my intention. She wasn't listening, as she was only listening to her own internal emotions. She keeps pressing me, and then asks why I get defensive when I refuse to say for the 3rd time that I would not do that to her. I got angry and said "you refuse to challenge these emotions, so now you are making me do it for you, and I'm not responsible for those feelings you have." Am I missing something here? I used to be able to handle these things without getting angry, but she just never stops until I get mad. She apologized, but does it really count if I can know like clockwork it will happen again in a few weeks? Feel like I'm going crazy.

Your best success is to wait until after the luteal phase and talk to her about her behavior.

Secondly, she does need to work through the trauma with her ex outside of the luteal phase. Underlying issues always exacerbate things and some CBT and other counselling will help her work through that problem so that then the luteal phase come it's less of a problem.

My girlfriend is a nutritionist who has started something called Seed Cycling to help her with her period, but won't see or talk to a psychiatrist or even try something like SSRIs. Is there hope?

BREAK THE CYCLE

In May, a few days before the PMDD extravaganza, I went to visit Tony where he was in New York City for work. The day was gorgeous, and I had a red dress on, but I fell into the darkest mood while we were eating at food carts in Flatiron. Blackness. I was in the red zone. We sat in Washington Square Park. The sun was annoying. The ice cream was annoying.

When I got back upstate, I started listening to therapist Esther Perel's podcast *Where Should We Begin?*, where she interviews anonymous couples who talk about their marital problems. The conversations are tough to stomach. While I listened, I anxiously took cans and boxes out of the pantry and reorganized everything. I kept telling Tony I couldn't go to the PMDD festival. I was too broke and felt too shitty. Fuck it. Fuck everything. (It was more of a conference than a festival, but I liked how it conjured images of a uterus piñata and red streamers.)

Tony Venmoed me some money to tide me over. He said I had to go to the conference and reminded me I'd been looking forward to it for months.

When the plane landed the next evening, we were stuck on the tarmac for hours because of a downpour. The flight attendant came on the PA system and angrily told whoever was vaping to stop vaping. Welcome to Boca Raton.

Tony had asked me how many people would be at the conference; I had no idea. I speculated about five hundred. There ended up being just eighty-four, significantly more than the eleven people who showed the first year.

May 16, 2018: Day 1 (Day 24 of cycling)

The PMDD mixer began at 6:00 p.m. in an event space in the lower level of the hotel. After carefully choosing my outfit, including on-sale floral pants from Anthropologie—which I hoped conveyed "I have PMDD, but I also have my shit together"—I took the elevator downstairs and entered the darkish dining room. I checked in and found the lanyard with my first name on it. They were selling merchandise: black backpacks that read FIGHT LIKE A PMDD GIRL, chakra bracelets, silver bracelets engraved with BE BRAVE, and a few books like *We Need to Talk About PMDD.*

I wasn't hungry, but I made a plate of crackers and veggies and fruit, and then went to the bar and ordered a tequila and soda with lime, which is something else I do for my acne, because tequila is supposedly the cleanest alcohol with the least sugar, and sugar can cause acne. It would be so nice to just eat and drink without having to consider acne.

I sat down next to two women, inviting myself into their conversation. One was the mother of a twenty-six-year-old woman with PMDD. The other was Katie Bigras, a nutritionist devoted to holistic PMDD tools. Katie was luminous, with almost-butt-length brown hair. There was something familiar about her. "As soon as I saw you, I *knew* we'd be friends," she said later. Slowly, more women joined us. There was Cynthia, a somatic therapist who lived in Denver and was attending with her mother, and another woman from Utah who was there with her girlfriend and her mother. Suddenly the table had grown from three to ten.

Katie explained that after figuring out her sweet spot of supplementation (calcium, 5-HTP, magnesium) and a lot of self-love, she'd had her PMDD mostly under control, but then described one of her recent meltdowns: she was at a family gathering and her toddler nephew looked her in the eye and said, "I don't like you," and she cried in her car for a couple hours.

"I can wake up in the morning and look out the same window and nothing has changed, but everything feels different," another woman said.

"We call it 'madface,'" her girlfriend added. "Oh, madface is here."

"This is pure indulgence," another woman said, "but does anyone notice any creativity surges during hell week?"

Someone at the table described PMDD as postpartum

depression every month. Others described it as two weeks in prison. I began feeling grateful that I only experienced symptoms for two to seven days.

It was curious to speak with these women. To see them as attractive, ambitious, articulate people, but to know they also go batshit, fly off the handle. I tried to guess who had PMDD. I was wrong most of the time. At one point, I spent twenty minutes speaking with a woman who ended up being a therapist without PMDD. Whenever someone confessed that they didn't have PMDD, my heart sank. *You are so lucky.*

Similarly, I was envious of people with different symptoms than mine. For example, I wished my symptoms were binge eating and depression as opposed to rage and paranoia. Other people probably wished their bloating and anxiety were replaced with anger and brain fog. Grass is always greener on the other PMDD side.

May 17, 2018: Day 2 (Day 25 of cycling)
We had to be in the lecture hall at 9:00 a.m. I spotted Katie immediately. She said, "I hope this isn't weird, but I saved you a seat."

First up was an older white male doctor, who basically told us that going on an antidepressant would eradicate our symptoms. Next, an expert in PMDD diagnosis explained that there is genetic testing that identifies women who carry the VAL and/or MTHFR (did anyone else think of this as motherfucker?) genes, which may make you predisposed to having PMDD.

A psychologist gave a lecture on DBT (dialectical behavioral therapy) and CBT (cognitive behavioral therapy), bringing their principles of "wise mind" and "reasonable mind" to "PMDD mind" (which is ruled by hot thoughts, emotions, feelings, urges). One CBT tool is called "opposite to emotion behavior": you identify the emotion (sadness), identify the mood-dependent behavior (inaction/isolation), and then do the opposite of that (exercise, social interaction, productive behavior). After a while, the feedback loop is broken. One of her suggestions for when you're angry, for example, was to "be a little nice" instead.

A woman in the front row raised her hand. "I don't agree with you. If I'm *mad* in my PMDD mind, I can't just *be a little nice*." She had PMDD symptoms for three weeks out of the month. I was so glad she spoke up; I happen to love both DBT and CBT—they helped me a lot in my twenties—but I knew it wasn't always possible to break the feedback loop of negative emotions in the moment. I wished someone would talk about how to deal with the rage.

Because I only went to college for two seconds, I never learned how to take notes. Sometimes in the writing classes I teach, I see people scribbling furiously or annotating whatever it is we are reading. I have never learned how to do that, and I have never taken notes on a computer. These are my notes from that day, transcribed from my notebook:

Light diffuser

Weighted blanket

Women w/ PMDD have a higher rate of past
psychiatric mood and anxiety

Comorbidity

2 out of 3 women with PMDD have history
w/ postpartum depression

Women with PMDD have more obsessive
personality traits

Take calcium

Do genetic testing

molecule by molecule

1:3 ratio

Women are more likely to attempt suicide,
but men are more likely to die b/c they
choose more lethal ways

Teresa Soutas: a wellness coach

*Abnormal response to normal hormone
changes*

Sensitivity to change

#Hormonesensitivity

PME = Premenstrual Exacerbation

Characteristics of Hormone Sensitive Females

Traumatic life events

Objective life stressors

Recent perceived stress

Impulsivity/emotion-related sensitivity

Trait impulsivity

VAL gene carriers

Higher brain has more difficulty controlling
   things

BPD could be chronic PMDD

Losing weight can affect hormone levels

Eat tryptophan—nuts, seeds, pistachios, pumpkin seeds, turkey, chicken, dark chocolate

Calcium/Vitamin D 1000mg a day

Chasteberry!!!!!!!!!!!!

Exercise in the luteal phase

Vitamin B6

20 jumping jacks

SSRI

Citalopram

Andrea Chisholm gynecologist—reach out
   to her for questions

Aromatherapy lamp—sage, lavender, colored
   lights + music

The day was long; at lunch I ducked out to pick up a prescription for an antibiotic for my cystic acne. I hadn't been on an

antibiotic in about a year, but that's how bad this cyst was. It made me self-conscious with everyone I spoke to. I considered skipping the latter half of the day but convinced myself I'd just get depressed.

One misconception of PMDD is that it is a hormone imbalance. But PMDD is not a hormone imbalance; it's an abnormal reaction to normal hormones. Your hormones are doing everything they're supposed to be doing: in the luteal phase, the two weeks leading up to your period after ovulation, progesterone rises and releases a chemical called allopregnanolone (my new favorite word, just *rolls off the tongue*), which in the majority of women makes them more subdued, fatigued, cranky. But some women are sort of allergic to the allopregnanolone, and their bodies perceive it as a threat.

We learned that three of the women on the board of directors ended up getting hysterectomies for their symptoms, which was disheartening to me. Two out of three of them had children and husbands. During pregnancy, PMDD symptoms disappear for most women, though if you have PMDD, you are more prone to experiencing postpartum depression.

Amanda LaFleur, one of the directors, described being on the thirtieth floor of a hotel with her husband and in-laws and feeling so disoriented that it was as though she was floating above the scene, watching herself change diapers. She told her husband she was having thoughts of throwing her newborn off the balcony because then she'd be able to sleep, and no one would need her anymore. Her outbursts were linked to her period, and the cyclical nature of symptoms mirrored the PMDD she'd experienced prepregnancy. She'd had symptoms since she was a teenager.

At the table flanking mine, I recognized Brett Buchert. She was sitting between her mother and father. She was the founder of the Me v PMDD app, where you can track your symptoms, use a self-care journal, find resources, and fight PMDD "like a warrior," as they say. Brett was twenty-two and was diagnosed with PMDD when she was twenty-one.

"Both of my parents have been a huge support to me in my journey," she told me. She'd created the app with her mom, Sheila.

She said she took an antidepressant called Viibryd, a medication called finasteride that prevents the conversion of progesterone to allopregnanolone, and a birth control pill called Tri-Lo-Sprintec. "I also take iron, vitamin B5, vitamin D, and a probiotic. It's quite a mix, but it's helped make my PMDD much more manageable."

Some women told me they keep ice packs in their car to use when they get symptomatic. Some use weighted blankets. Some use a scent diffuser that blows lavender oil while changing colors. One woman, married for fourteen years, locks herself in a hotel room to rage-write in her journal for a couple days. She attended the conference with her husband; I admired their relationship.

The last workshop of the night was called PMDD Date Night, led by sex therapist and mental health counselor Chasity Chandler. She specialized in LGBT relationships, trauma, and substance abuse. She was the only one at the conference who addressed PMDD in transmasculine people and trans men.

Chasity said something that has haunted me since: "It sounds like a lot of you have supportive partners. Who supports the supportive partner? Often the PMDD-er knows exactly what they want and need. When was the last time you asked your partner what they needed?"

She declared that date nights don't need to happen at night. They can be date brunches, date walks, date afternoons. She suggested taking turns to plan one-hour, in-home date nights, and to never use dates for talking about your relationship. She suggested having two jars: one with ideas for a high-energy date night, for when the PMDD-er is in the follicular phase, and others for a low-energy date night, when they are in the luteal phase.

One woman dating a woman with PMDD said she wished she had a PMDD support group. She said it is unusual to be in a relationship where someone loves you and thinks you're the greatest thing ever and then one day they just hate you. "The hardest part for me is, being a logical person, not being able to reason with her, though she was so reasonable the day before."

"One of my clients spent ten thousand dollars on a divorce

lawyer while she was in one of those episodes," Chasity said. "No joke. Seriously."

This workshop made me so sympathetic toward Tony. I wished he was there.

Notes from Chasity's lecture:

We are wired for vulnerability

If we want everyone else to be vulnerable, why can't we be?

"If we share our story with someone who has empathy, shame does not exist"

Who supports the supportive partner???

Who takes care of the caregiver?

Make a game plan for the Week

Written out protocol

Ask: Is this a real issue? Or just a PMDD issue?

Persona Play

Overcommunication

Partner can regulate you by being nonreactive

Come up with a new language

Man in the audience says he would like to be able to take a pill to feel what PMDD is like for just one hour.

BE INTENTIONAL about a date.

The Rock Conversation. Each person gets

turn with the rock. Hold the rock and say:
3 things you're grateful for, something on
your heart, something you're looking forward to
Emotional nakedness is what we need for
desire.
Mental health + sexual health is part of
physical health.

I went back to my room and passed the fuck out.

May 18, 2018: Day 3 (Day 26 of cycling)
Well, shit. I woke up with full-blown PMDD. The shakiness.
The feeling that all blood has drained from your face. The urge
to bawl over nothing (everything) and sleep.

I'd been worried this would happen. Having PMDD at a
PMDD conference was like falling asleep at a narcolepsy conference. I was cranky and anxious, and my heart was beating
quickly as soon as I opened my eyes. My skin was inflamed,
red, and breaking out. I decided to let myself sleep in and miss
the morning lectures on suicidal ideation.

I was in tears over . . . nothing. But for me, having tears over
nothing was a good sign. In the past, my tears came out as rage
and blame, and I projected those emotions onto Tony. It was
huge for me to realize I was just sad and edgy because I was
going to get my period any day.

Tony and I spoke on the phone to say good morning, and I felt my sensitivity coming on. On another day, his tone of voice wouldn't be an issue, but on Day 26 of my cycle, it felt like the world was falling apart. (I mean, it kind of was.) I was up for a fight, and I was going to *win*.

Tony and I have made a deal that, through our travels, we won't (I won't) text thoughts that should be saved for bigger conversations to have in person. But when my PMDD acts up, this all goes out the window because I love a good text evisceration. In PMDD brain, I ruminate on anything he's ever said that has irked me and tell him about them. When I started doing this in my hotel room, Tony texted me back, "STOP," along with the red stop sign emoji and a Bitmoji of him as a cartoon character getting hit with a bomb.

I decided to go eat breakfast alone, ignoring my phone. I ordered a coffee and an oatmeal skillet. The waitress was trying to chat with me about the book I was reading, and it made me emotional. I went to cry in the bathroom.

Laura saw me there and asked if I was okay. I said I was but that I needed a little time. Her tote bag read BE KINDER TO YOUR VAGINA.

"Yeah," she said. "That was pretty triggering for everyone."

I felt dishonest that I was only triggered by my hormones, not the suicidal ideation lecture I'd skipped. I felt like a liar for not admitting I hadn't gone.

Upstairs at the lecture hall, I saw Amanda and Laura and

was greeted with such love. Amanda has the most insanely gorgeous smile I've ever seen in my life, and I burst into tears when she hugged me.

Sometimes all it takes is someone asking you if you're okay. Amanda said that something they were trying to do for the next year was have a room of peer support counselors for this exact situation.

It was funny to be around women who were so well versed in PMDD language. "I'm cycling" was a phrase I'd never heard before that I began hearing everywhere.

"Sorry, I get chatty when I am in the luteal phase," Katie said. Until three months ago I'd never even heard of the luteal phase.

"I'm on that day of my cycle where you can't sit still," someone in the elevator told me.

"What day is that?" I asked.

"Twenty-one."

"I'm on twenty-six," I said.

Some people were popping 5-HTP and avoiding gluten and others were saying they can easily avoid gluten and dairy and eat a bunch of kale until they're in the luteal phase, when they'd order big cheeseburgers. There were women with dark chocolate in their purses; I asked for a piece from one of them. Some women were cranky because sleeping in dry hotel rooms is hard, and rooming with their mothers is also hard. Some women had aromatherapy oils they passed around for the rest of us to rub on our wrists. Some women were vocal about needing more caffeine. Some women were pregnant. All women were cycling.

Amanda and Laura told me to take an Uber to the beach, put my feet in the ocean, walk on the sand. I didn't want to go that far, literally and metaphorically, but I did change into my favorite long pink dress, bought some sunscreen out of the vending machine, and lay by the pool listening to Shakira's album *Laundry Service*, which I've recently figured out does wonders for my mood. (Don't ask—I don't know.) Tony called and we had a talk, which didn't go awesome, but we've had worse. We got out of the hole successfully and I went into my first lecture of the day. I didn't want to miss Jenni Kay Long, who was presenting a lecture called Navigating PMDD with Mindfulness.

Jenni Kay Long is a therapist in Denver with PMDD. Her PMDD symptoms began at age twelve, and her panic was so debilitating she couldn't walk from her bedroom to the bathroom without fainting. In her twenties, she was going to yoga five times a week to manage symptoms, and going to acupuncture and talk therapy. The number of days she had symptoms each month began to shrink, going from two weeks a month to one week, then to three days. She was passionate about helping others with PMDD, so she got her yoga teacher training certificate, her acupuncture license, her social work degree. "That's what all those ridiculous letters after my name are," she explained. "I wanted to get all of the things for myself that had helped me." She was pregnant with her second child and had one of the sweetest speaking voices I'd ever heard.

"Every symptom you have is a need that isn't being met," she said. For example, you could be experiencing heavy cramps because you are lacking magnesium. You could be experiencing hyperarousal and panic, which are caused by a dip in estrogen and marked increase in progesterone in the days leading up to your period—and which can combine with a not-fully-healed trauma from your childhood to become impulsivity, hypervigilance, defensiveness, feeling unsafe, reactive, angry, and having racing thoughts. This is why, she explained, a layered and holistic treatment approach to PMDD is most effective.

From Acupuncture to Zoloft, A–Z Treatments for PMDD was the final panel. Toward the end of it, a woman from the audience raised her hand and said, "There is absolutely hope. I never thought I'd find someone because I try to talk him out of being in a relationship with me all the time. He continually tells me, 'Hey, you're worth it.' So, there *are* people who see us—the *true* us. So don't let our disease or condition deter you from trying to have a meaningful relationship, because for me that's part of the healing, and love is the antidote to shame." The rest of us applauded.

450 periods = 6 years of being symptomatic

Burden to manage symptoms

"Each symptom is a need that is not being met." —Jenni Kay Long

When a trauma happens, attachment is broken.

Re-building secure attachment.

Hyperarousal—overwhelm, panic, impulsivity, hyper-vigilant, defensiveness, feeling unsafe, reactive, angry, racing thoughts

Luteal Phase:

Crisis management

Debrief the week

Body-based skills

Follicular Phase:

Reflection

Go deeper

Work towards long term goals.

Treatments:

Psychotherapy

Education

Lifestyle Planning

Accuwellness
Trauma-sensitive yoga
Mindfulness Skills Training
"Val Gene"
"MTHFR Gene"

My writing workshop was the last session of the conference:
7:00 p.m. I was too tired and drained to be nervous about teaching. I didn't do a PowerPoint or use the whiteboard, but I used
the microphone. I read from my personal essays about PMDD,
which was interesting—to give a reading about something so
specific to people who experience the same exact symptoms.

In the creative nonfiction classes I teach, I do a prompt
called I Remember, taken from Joe Brainard's 1970 memoir of
the same name. In the book, Brainard begins every sentence
with "I remember"—a nonchronological detailed account of
his coming-of-age. Usually in my classes, I have the students
do an I Remember about anything they want, but that night
the assignment was specific: Write an I Remember about your
first period. Even if you don't really remember. Even if it's hard.
Even if it hurts.

Sometimes I'll get a class where no one wants to read their
work. This drastically changes the dynamic, not to mention the
lesson plan. In a class where no one offers to read and everyone is timid, I'll have so much extra time unaccounted for. But
that night, almost everyone wanted to read. They passed the

microphone around with gusto and spoke confidently, expres-
sively. Some people choked up; some laughed. Although I've
been teaching memoir writing for three years, and although it
is not a competition, this was one of the more moving nights
in my life.

Because everyone wanted to read their work, we didn't
get to the other prompts I'd planned: Write a letter to your
PMDD self from the perspective of your higher self. Write a
letter to someone you've hurt while in PMDD brain. Make a
list of tools you can use for the next time you're experiencing
full-blown PMDD.

I skipped all of those for time's sake and pulled out
self-compassion cards, handing them out until everyone had
one. I'd purchased them for Tony for Christmas, but maybe I'd
actually bought them for me. I had packed them in my suitcase
at the last minute. The cards read things like: *What wish would
you make for your teenage self? Consider one of your role models.
What are three things you have in common with them as a human
being? Is part of your body calling out in pain or discomfort? Can
you just be with it without trying to change it for five breaths?*

Afterward, people came up to me and told me how powerful my workshop was. It was a revelation—a "growth spurt"
I called it later, when talking with Tony on the phone—to
realize I can be struggling yet still help those who struggle.
Simultaneously.

Do you ever have those times when you feel you are exactly

where you're supposed to be? They come around a few times a year for me, more if I'm lucky. Those times you feel good in your body, no FOMO, grounded, loved, and loving. The moment you know you are on the right path. That's what happened to me that night, post-workshop.

A bunch of us went into the hot tub and drank tequila and wine and talked until after midnight. I went to bed first, and Katie, whom I gave my extra bed to, came to the room an hour later. We talked until we fell asleep, like old friends.

At around 5:00 a.m. the hotel's fire alarm went off and we all groggily walked outside to the front of the hotel until staff confirmed it was a false alarm. It was fitting, after the level of intimacy we'd achieved over three days, to see everyone stripped down with naked faces, eye masks, flip-flops, robes, and boxer shorts.

May 19, 2018: Day 4 (Day 27 of cycling)
There's a quote I heard once: not everything can be healed or cured, but it should be properly named.

Because of our sexist culture, there is a constant little voice in my head telling me I'm just "crazy." There are men who think that PMDD is an "excuse to act bitchy," and there's intense cultural stigma around "period brain." Each month after PMDD passes for me, I question if I was just being dramatic, and tell myself that next month I'll be able to control it.

Many of the women I met described sitting in dozens of

skeptical doctors' offices before they made it to the conference. Even the specialists presenting were only speculating about PMDD causes and treatments; it is nearly impossible to figure out what prompts each unique symptom in each woman's unique body.

But in Boca Raton, for three days, we were all seen, heard, and believed. *Whatever they're experiencing, they're experiencing.*

On the plane, I pulled up the voice memos I'd recorded. Jenni Kay, Chasity, Amanda. I put on my headphones and listened to their stories, their tips, their points of view. I buckled my seat belt and turned the volume all the way up.

When I got off the plane, I had a voice mail from my doctor, who said my blood results came back low on iron, magnesium, iodine, and zinc, with a suggestion of which supplements to purchase to help with the fainting. "Drink Gatorade," she said, "and eat meat for breakfast."

Back at my apartment, Tony and his daughter had a WEL-COME HOME sign and bouquet of flowers on the counter. My favorite pizza was in the oven. My laundry was done and folded. The three of us cuddled together on the small yellow couch and watched *Back to the Future Part II*. And in the morning—because it is the punctuation of my life—I woke up with my period.

THE BENCH

The idea to propose to Tony came to me on a mundane June afternoon. I was by myself; Tony and Sadie were at Zoom Flume Water Park and would return in the evening. This notion was so fierce I didn't second-guess it and immediately began looking for nontraditional rings. I quickly found the perfect handmade titanium-and-lapis ring and ordered it a few days later, because I'd unexpectedly received a hefty royalty check. My plan was to bring the ring with me on our vacation to Portugal and Spain in September, our first time leaving the country together.

But I ended up bringing the ring everywhere that summer. I brought it to Cape Cod, just in case, when we were camping with my family. I brought it on another trip to Madison, Wisconsin, visiting Tony's family.

The ring became an emblem for any interaction, negative or positive, between us. If we were having an argument, I fantasized about grabbing the ring and saying, "I even got you a ring, asshole!" and throwing it. If I was anxious, I'd worry that the ring was unattractive, the wrong size, sure that he'd hate the blue lapis, and what a pity it would be when he went to put it on, and it didn't fit.

This cyclical behavior can break even the strongest of bonds.

I tried pushing her sentence out of my mind.

I phoned a close friend, who told me she'd also proposed. How hadn't I known that? Maybe I *had* known, but in my single days, I just hadn't cared. What were the odds? She was one of my best friends, whom I'd traveled all over with for years. I didn't know anyone else who had. "I knelt in the snow with two engraved rings when we were walking our dogs one night. They were engraved with 'love of my life.'"

Shit—my ring wasn't engraved. And I only had one ring. I asked another friend: "Should I have two rings?"

"I think you can do whatever the hell you want, you know?" she said.

I called some jewelers, but since the ring was titanium and not silver, engraving was an expensive hassle. "You have your whole life to get them engraved," my therapist said, calming me down.

Of course I wanted to marry him. He'd once said to me, "I love the dark parts of you." I'd be an idiot not to propose.

✦

I'd decided to go off Prozac because after the PMDD extravaganza, one day before my period, I'd thrown some water from a glass toward Tony during an episode. My logic (which you could definitely poke a hole in) was that if I was still throwing cups of water at people, the Prozac wasn't working.

Prozac is said to have a long half-life. This would explain why going off in June didn't affect me until August, when life suddenly felt heavy and small tasks too hard. In August, I began waking up wounded and tearful. The day of my worst cramps I spent in our bedroom, drawing the deep-red curtains shut. Having your period in the East Coast cruel humidity of August should be illegal.

"Look at the bedroom," I said to Tony at the end of the day.

"It looks insane in there."

There were a dozen mugs and glasses, bottles of ibuprofen and THC salve. Tony's crumpled tissues. A red hot-water bottle, half a dozen books scattering the bed.

The days were ninety-nine degrees with 96 percent humidity. I bled and cramped like I'd never bled and cramped before. Tony was having allergy attacks and couldn't breathe; I was waking up terrified of the day.

August turned to September, and PMDD trickled on. I was attending a weeklong writing workshop by Carole Maso at the Millay Colony, and on the first day, I realized what might be going wrong in this book. One of the first things Carole said was to write from an altered state. PMDD is my altered state, but it is so altered that when I'm in it, I don't do anything, or I don't remember what I do.

I remember texting my friend Diana Spechler, a writer who also struggles with PMDD, from bed, sobbing. Diana, I knew, would get it, as she had written a column for *The New York Times* called Going Off where she tapered off her medications in real time. One line from the final column in the series had stuck with me: "The goal is to feel O.K., not to prove that you are O.K. without meds."

"Can you write when you're in this?" she texted back.

"I probably could but I never feel motivated to, or to try."

"It could help, but also, nothing helps," she kindly responded.

"Right."

Being in the throes of emotion, stuck in a PMDD episode, I'm likely yelling, crying, sleeping, or throwing something. The last thing I'd ever think to do is sit down and work on a book. But I wondered if the book suffered because of that. I'd once had the idea to force myself to write during PMDD symptoms, but PMDD laughs in the face of my creative plans. Women are told to channel their rage into art, but come on, people.

In Carole's class, we went around the table describing what we were working on. I said I was writing about a year in the life of a period. The person next to me misunderstood. "I thought you meant you were writing from the period's perspective."

"I wish that's what I meant," I said.

If I did have swaths of during-PMDD writing, would I even want to share it in this book? In the class, we go on and on about how our memoirs aren't our diaries, and god knows they aren't. The structure to this memoir has been moved around and manipulated at least eighty-five times to be crafted into something marketable, sellable, readable. How could I possibly get the swirling unknowable ephemeral capricious rage down on the page while maintaining a linear, organized book? And does the book suffer because I cannot? Because I do not?

Labor Day weekend, and our assignment for the workshop is to go to the Columbia County Fair, a fair I'd grown up going to, a fair I'd been avoiding. We were supposed to choose a spot to sit and write for three hours. I was in that fatigued state that happens after three days of the blood. Relieved it's over, but feeling weak and melancholy. I felt defeated from fighting, defeated by my period, defeated by the writing prompt.

✦

On a pale yellow bench in front of an even paler yellow building, two girls sit to my right. One eats popcorn out of a red box while the other looks at her phone. I can't pinpoint exactly when I stopped liking, or started disliking, fairs, zoos, or "organized fun," as I call it. Age twelve? Twenty? Did it happen slowly and then all at once?

The girls are discussing how skinny someone is. "She's got no food in her," they say. I don't see who they're talking about—I looked up too late.

I ordered a strawberry-banana smoothie and now I want a soft pretzel. I see the fake cheese is a dollar extra and I want that, too. I always get pretzels when I'm at either malls or fairs, which is about once a year.

The girls are gone, have left me. It's been said that writing in public scares people. Or that you look insane. I forget. Going to get a pretzel now.

When I got up to throw the rest of my smoothie away, I have a text from my dad: *Sharece just saw Katie Holmes at the fair.* (I don't know how to respond, then forget to.)

Ate my pretzel, didn't regret it.

The man who sold it to me called me "sweetie" twice and "hon" once.

Another man said, "Heyyyy, Cindy Crawford," as I walked by, showing his age. I was disgusted, and also it was the nicest thing anyone has said to me in weeks. Tony and I have been arguing so much. It starts as soon as we wake up and are in the kitchen.

My yellow bench is all filled up with people now.

I moved to a green bench and the same two girls from earlier are on it.

"What's my favorite pizza?" one asks.

"Bacon."

"Candy?"

"KitKat."

"Fruit?"

"Mango. "

"Place to go shopping?"

"Macy's."

One of the girls' little sisters tries to tell the older girls something, and the older one looks up at her: "WE'RE HAVING A CONVERSATION!"

The younger one shrinks back, says, "I'm sorry . . . I didn't know."

On the phone with his brother, Tony mentioned I was sick with cramps. His brother told Tony about a memory of a time he was at a Halloween party and had really bad stomach cramps, which put him in a bad mood.

Tony told me and I spat back, "Those kinds of cramps are *completely* different from menstrual cramps."

In retrospect, though, it has been the only time a man has tried to relate to my cramps, instead of alienating me further. He could have said, "That sucks for her," or complained about his own girlfriend and her time of the month. But he met my misery with his own misery, and with empathy and compassion. I look at it now as maybe the nicest thing that's ever been said to me by a male about my period.

◆

What if he said no? How could I propose after this hellish August? I couldn't imagine him saying no, but I couldn't imagine *anything*. It was a situation you could not be prepared for—the ultimate free fall. It felt like exposure therapy—doing what I was most afraid of. Some people catastrophize airplanes, elevators, and public speaking. I catastrophize marriage.

What if he said, "I'm touched but I want to work on the relationship more first"? That would be a valid answer. I've known friends whose partners didn't want to get married until their finances were in order, or they were making more money. Tony saying no wouldn't be the craziest thing that ever happened.

What if he said, "I'm not sure I can be married to someone with PMDD"?

I mean, I could see he was crazy about me. And I'd never met a man I could even go to the grocery store with. (The intimacy of their seeing what I eat was uncomfortable). Could I really have a *Story of a Happy Marriage*, to quote Ann Patchett, even if my parents didn't?

We went to therapy together, which I had to look at as progress instead of a failure.

"I'm not going anywhere," Tony said.

"He's right here, working things out with you," my therapist said.

Slowly I realized that the nightmare month didn't mean we had to break up. It meant we were able to stay together.

On the television show *Couples Therapy*, psychoanalyst Dr. Orna Guralnik said: "You have to let go of your childhood when you're creating a new family. Are you just gonna repeat what has been handed to you? Are you just gonna repeat the mistakes your parents made? Or are you going to be able to kind of jump the fence and do something different?"

I was jumping the fence.

✦

I went back on ten milligrams of Prozac before our trip. If I didn't have to suffer so badly, why should I? I decided to think of it as a really good vitamin. I remembered Sheila calling it "a little bit of sunshine."

The ring was packed in my floral carry-on suitcase, hidden among my T.J.Maxx jumpsuits.

I read that when couples argue, they should be standing or sitting at the same level. One should never be standing over the other. We took this tip into consideration whenever we were arguing. Planning my proposal, I knew there was no way I'd get down on one knee, which seemed embarrassing. We'd be eye to eye. Relatedly, Tony read in *The Psychology of Trading* by Brett N. Steenbarger about a theory where if you're fighting with your significant other, you can fight as much as you want to so long as you go into the closet together and stand on one foot.

On our first full day in Lisbon, we were jet-lagged and giddy. The Alfama district where we were staying was all cobblestones and hills. That night, we got dressed up and took photos of each other in front of muraled walls on our walk to dinner. I remember thinking, This will be the last photo of me as a non-engaged woman. My expression looks happy and a little afraid.

After reading about restaurants with "the best sunset view in Lisbon," I had three restaurant ideas. The first one was closed, the second was full, and the final one didn't look good to us. We'd walked a few miles out of the way by this time and I felt dumb. Finally, we found a hole-in-the-wall that was romantic, and while we ate our cod and olives, we listened to live fado music as the lights turned down. Across from me Tony kept telling me he loved me, and I considered handing the ring to him in the dark restaurant. But I had another rule for my proposal: I wanted us to be outside.

At around 10:30 p.m., we were walking home through a little courtyard that had tiled buildings, potted plants, and one orange tree poking out of a square in the pavement. Tony was about to go down a long, narrow staircase, and I knew if I didn't do it now, I never would. At the last possible second before his foot hit the stairs, I said, "Let's sit on this bench for a minute. When do you get to sit on a tiled bench?"

Nerves. Heart flutters. Adrenaline.

"Why don't you smoke a cigarette?" I said, normally not a fan of his casual smoking.

He lit up, and I handed him my phone.

"Will you read this thing I wrote today?"

He began reading at what seemed like a fast pace. He was smiling. He said, "Oh my god," once and then kept repeating it at louder and more intense volumes. His body started to shake, and mine shook in response. He was crying, and I was crying the most joyful cry I've ever cried. I felt more empowered and alive in that moment than ever before. Still shaking, we walked to our Airbnb, and uncorked a bottle of red. Tony called his parents and then my mom, saying, "Your daughter just proposed to me."

Proposing was a new feeling. It made me feel high. I was taking control of my life. Making decisions based on stability, growth, and risk, instead of making decisions out of impulsivity and fear.

The next evening we found a tiny speakeasy called Ulysses, and spent a while talking with the owner and bartender. He was impressed that I ordered fernet, and even though he didn't know anything about me and how relevant this detail was to me, he went on to explain that fernet is helpful for menstrual cramps. Tony and I looked at each other and smiled. We'd chosen the right bar.

✦

In my midtwenties, when I used to cat-sit, dog-sit, babysit, and house-sit for somewhere free to live, I'd constantly read memoirs by women. As a single person, I felt so deceived and abandoned when they ended with getting married. Books I loved did this. *Loose Girl* by Kerry Cohen. *The Chronology of Water* by Lidia Yuknavitch. Cheryl Strayed doesn't get married at the end of *Wild*, but she alludes to it, and will.

Those books had been *my* story, and then in the last few pages they weren't anymore.

I feel bad about having the marriage proposal in my book because I remember those house-sitting days: lounging around, having way too much time on my hands, having affairs, day-drinking, aimlessly walking around, reading a book and throwing it off the bed when the female narrator got married. Sadie likes telling people about the scene in Greta Gerwig's *Little Women*, how the publisher tells Jo the narrator has to be either married or dead at the end.

✦

A week after my proposal, Tony looked me in the eye and told me what I'd done was very brave. We were in a cab driving from downtown Barcelona to the airport. We held hands, his now adorned with the lapis ring, and my fingers, plain, feeling full of opportunity. On the radio, "Ironic" by Alanis Morissette was playing.

When we landed back in the States, cranky after our eight-hour flight that served zero food, we got into a trite argument, first about what kind of food to order, and then, when we got back our apartment, another about where the weird, rotten smell was coming from. It felt *exactly* like coming home.

PART FIVE

THE RING

Four months after we were engaged, shit got weird. Thanksgiving through New Year's was a complete blur. Tony's parents had come to visit for Christmas, and his dad ended up in the hospital. There was a lot of self-medicating with weed and alcohol. Tony did something out of character that triggered my trust issues, and over brunch for his birthday, he was asked to join an eight-week tour of Europe and Lebanon that got extended past my birthday in April. This was the longest (plus unplanned and short notice) amount of time we'd ever been apart. Without physical touch, we'd be relying on technology for communication, and that was one of our triggers for fighting.

Although our industries and careers are totally different, I gave in to the temptation of comparing them. He was playing venues for thousands of people in places like Spain, Finland, Slovakia, Germany, and Denmark with a group of successful and sickeningly talented singers and musicians. I was jealous as I sat at home writing about my period. I'd been doing this for three years at that point, and even my own agent at the time rarely responded to me until she eventually admitted she didn't have a vision for my book. I felt like a loser. A PMDD-having, period-writing loser. My grandmother had passed away, I was burned out from the hustle of freelance teaching for little money and the responsibilities of being a parent while my partner was gone. It was a dark time; meanwhile, I was sending wedding invitations out. There was a day I was supposed to go with my mom to a local shop to choose stuff for a bridal shower, but I was too depressed and spent the day in bed. With a seven-hour time difference between us, it felt almost impossible to connect.

We used the Marco Polo app, I went to group therapy that Anna had, and we decided to read the book *Mating in Captivity* by Esther Perel at the same time to stay connected and email our thoughts on the book. Instead of emails about the book, though, we ended up in PMDD-induced phone calls, and then follow-up emails in the PMDD aftermath.

> Tony: I spent hours upon hours with you in PMDD and you destroying me while I paced the streets of Glasgow and I have a very short tolerance for that right now. You were

accusing me of lying while I was taking a shit and thinking that I sent you a false picture. Your mind is making things into things that are not. I have multiple times, over and over and over told you this and it feels nearly impossible for you to take it in. Maybe when you get your period and your hormones return you will be able to see that.

Chloe: I'm so so sorry PMDD took over our bond this week. Normally, I feel I've shrunk the symptoms to just a couple days but this week felt like a straight WEEK of PMDD. As you know, and I am so sorry for hurting you. It's fucking HARD you being gone for two months totally unplanned. I'll be sure to set up the calendar with alerts for next month. I am ashamed of how much darkness is coming up for me.

Tony: We've weathered some difficult and challenging storms and I think ultimately only strengthens our bond with each other. We can live a great life together and have been in so many ways. We need to treat each other with loving kindness. When

we're upset, find what it is and speak from
the heart, not the head. If it continues I can't
do that and will not play that game. No one
deserves that, especially your partner and I
know you intellectually know that. I need
your actions to start backing it up. I need
you to know that you are my love and only
you. Stop comparing and judging. It is a
waste of energy and time and is immature
and I'm tired of you bringing on something
else to create a story about to validate your
fears and anxieties.

When Tony's tour got extended even longer, he decided to fly
me to meet him in Beirut at the end of the tour in mid-April for
a belated birthday gift.

◆

While Tony was on tour during February and March, I used
my phone tons more than when he was home, and I developed
a Poshmark addiction. I purchased gold Kate Spade heels,
red Lotta clogs, brown MAC eyeshadow, and Betsey Johnson
heart-patterned pajamas. Everything fit and it felt like magic.
I sold stuff, too, but didn't make much money because I used
that money to buy stuff for myself.

A few nights before my period arrived, I was lying on the couch losing my life to hours on Poshmark. I realized a woman suspiciously named Sarah Jones had never shipped the shirt I ordered.

On Poshmark, you're supposed to ship stuff in two to five days. If it hasn't shipped in seven days, the buyer can cancel the order and get refunded. Every other day I'd asked Sarah Jones if she'd shipped my shirt. She'd only responded once and said it was going in the mail. I began reading the comments underneath her Meet the Posher page, and saw that someone else had had a similar problem. This woman was supposed to do a trade with Sarah. Instead of sending what she'd promised the woman, Sarah had kept the garment and never responded. I read the saddest comment I've maybe ever read on the internet: "You seemed like a nice girl," the woman wrote.

I was livid and barraged Sarah's page with comments, warning others about her. I forgot all about it, until I received this email a few weeks later:

Hello Chloe,

We here at Poshmark HQ truly value you as a member of the Poshmark community. This is why we are contacting you today about some activity from your account that is in violation of our guidelines.

In your time on Poshmark, we have noticed some behavior that violates our Community Guidelines. We require all Poshers to conduct themselves in a professional and trustworthy manner. We ask that you be respectful of others and follow Poshmark's community guidelines, or we may be forced to take action on your account.

What? I responded. *What did I do?*

Hi Chloe,

Thank you for reaching out to us. Your buying and selling privileges have been disabled for the following:

—Behaving in a manner that violates Community Guidelines

"This person is a total unethical a-hole. do not purchase anything from them unless you want to lose money. you suck, Sarah."

"Warning: This is a fake account. Do not

buy from this fraud. They don't ship their
purchases.

They will steal your money. Eff you Sarah"

I have to admit: when I saw what I'd written during a
PMDD brownout, I laughed. PMDD for once had come out at
a Postmark chick, instead of my fiancé.

◆

In Beirut, Tony and I walked around the city at sunset and listened to prayers. We were delighted to see each other, and I had
remorse for how the tour had gone. We got tattoos on our wrists.
We ate tabbouleh and flatbread ravenously. I saw women thread-
ing their daughters' mustaches and eyebrows on the street. We
visited the mosques—I wore a hijab and sat on the floor to pray.

One day we took a cooking class, and Tony and I were
talking to a woman who asked me what I was working on, and
I told her a book about PMDD.

"I think my nanny has that!" she said and went on to shit-
talk her nanny.

She said that when her nanny had her period, she became
a different person, and that sometimes she found drips of her
nanny's blood on the bathroom floor.

She said that once, before a party, she asked her nanny to replace the dying flowers throughout the house with fresh flowers. When the woman returned home, she found that the nanny had done the opposite: placed the dead flowers all around and thrown away the fresh ones.

To me, this anecdote represents PMDD more accurately than anything I've read. When you're in the darkness you cannot even tell the dead from the living.

✦

We were staying at a hostel called Grand Meshmosh in Gemmayzeh, near a ton of restaurants, shops, and a contemporary art museum called Sursock. Tony had purchased a tour of Byblos for that Saturday morning. Byblos is one of the oldest cities in the world, first inhabited between 8800 and 7000 B.C. Tony told me the Bible was written there.

I wasn't crazy pumped for the tour. I was actually sort of pissed, because this was my birthday present. My ideal way to get to know a city is by wandering in and out of cafés, parks, bookstores, bars, restaurants, and the rare museum. We'd traveled together before and are normally on the same page. But this tour was important to him and he'd been looking forward to it.

We had to meet our shuttle at 7:45 a.m. I had my heart set on coffee for the road, but nothing was open. We got into the car with two men who didn't speak to us. A few miles later, we pulled up to another hotel to pick up another traveler, and as she came into view, I had a strange, fleeting sensation I couldn't place. I liked her style—but wait, did I like it, or did it remind me of someone? Before I could figure it out, Tony said, "Woahhhhhh. That woman looks exactly like you." We both had curly hair, were wearing floral jumpsuits, high-tops, denim jackets, and aviators. We both even had tattoos on our wrists and delicate gold necklaces around our necks. We both wore leather backpacks. Tony and I cracked up as she got in the back seat with us. She told us she was from Turkey.

Before Byblos, the tour stopped at Jeita Grotto, a cave discovered in 1836. The stones all looked phallic and like they were wet with semen. If you want more description of the grotto and of *Our Lady of Lebanon* and all the other shit we saw, you should put down this book and go pick up a history book, because you will be disappointed.

I was hungry. Neither of us knew the tour was going to be eight hours, or guided. The grotto's "restaurant" only had ice cream and Snickers. Tony and I both had Snickers for breakfast.

In the upper cave, they split us into groups of six and put us in boats. There were no phones allowed—we had to put them in lockers—but I took mine with me. We snuck a video, which was also anticlimactic.

Afterward, I went to the bathroom and when I glanced

into the stall, I saw a hole in the floor to piss in. I had the dumbest possible outfit on—a jumpsuit. And not just a jumpsuit with zippers, but one with three buttons on top of my left shoulder that I'd have to undo. And then to get back into it, I'd have to pull some weird double-jointed contortionist shit. Fuck it, I thought. I'll hold it. Rather be uncomfortable holding my pee than get piss all over my clothing for the rest of this long day.

Normally I can't fall asleep so easily, but on the bus to Byblos I passed out hard on Tony's shoulder. Tony was obsessing about the guy sitting in front of us because he looked like Gru, the leader of the minions in *Despicable Me*. So we had my doppelgänger along with Gru for entertainment.

Our tour guide was a woman with a soft voice who wore a key around her neck. At Byblos she told us we had an hour to explore, that we'd then meet back up to visit a museum and castle. Tony and I walked through a magical field of yellow flowers and stones and took in the view. There was this little shack, and we joked the Bible was maybe written in it. We sat in there awhile, talking.

"I vow to never take you on a walking history tour again," he said.

"Thank god," I said.

"I vow to keep working on PMDD, especially when we're apart because of work," I said.

My Turkish sister, as we called her, was our landmark for

our tour group. Though we didn't speak more than twenty words to her, we'd excitedly say, "There's Sarah," when we spotted her.

The lunch was copious amounts of hummus and pita bread and tabbouleh and grilled meats. Our tour took up three large tables, and our table was quiet. Gru sat directly across from me and it was hard to keep my shit together. When I went upstairs to the bathroom, I heard one woman say to another, "This really makes you appreciate what you have at home." I wasn't sure if she meant the small bathrooms, which were fine, or the bus, or Lebanon, or what.

The awkwardness at the table got to be too much for me so I went outside to the Mediterranean Sea. Tony followed me and we took off our shoes and socks and splashed around, collected rocks. We sat on the beach in silence for a while, our legs dangling off the wall. My shoulders were burning from the sun.

"I vow to travel the world with you," Tony said.

We vowed some more, staring at the Mediterranean, and it was obvious to both of us that this was the best part of the day so far.

Leaving lunch, I said, "I miss Sarah."

"Me, too."

A quick bus ride to Harissa to see the Virgin Mary. We waited in line for twenty minutes and then took a zip line over Byblos, which made my hands sweat and feel panicked. What if there was a freak accident? At the top, we climbed the stairs to the statue. It was crowded and I was starting to get really bored. We took a bunch of selfies. I look tired in them. On the bus home, we were exhausted and bickered about something stupid. I moved seats and we sat across the aisle from each other, not speaking. We walked back toward our hotel in silence.

"I'm going to take some space for twenty-five minutes," I said. "I need to be alone after being in that herd of people."

Tony went back to the hostel and I walked down the street toward the bookstore that served wine. On my way, I stopped in a boutique jewelry store. The kid working there was in his early twenties and eating lunch. I told him it smelled good. He was wearing jeans with a white T-shirt that read HOLLISTER, CALIFORNIA in red. He pulled out a bunch of rings for me to look at. All unique, and if any had fit me, I would have bought one, but I'm a ring size four and all the rings were sevens and eights.

I'd been having a hard time finding a wedding ring. My birthstone is diamond, and I've always hated how they look on my pale skin. Maybe I was influenced by my mom, who had never worn a diamond. Diamonds seemed so basic, and a plain gold band seemed too boring. I wanted something interesting enough to be a conversation piece, but chill enough that I could wear it every day. I didn't want something so nice that I'd have to take off when I was doing the dishes. (Domestic queen, much?)

We'd done everything backward: I proposed to Tony with the perfect ring but didn't know how to find the equivalent for myself. I asked the kid when the store closed, and he told me 10:00 p.m. I said I'd come back with my fiancé. "I'll be waiting for you," he said.

✦

Tony and I met back up after my glass of white wine and reading time and went to find some dinner. We walked past the jewelry shop again, and I brought Tony in to show him. (Tony is into jewelry, something I love about him.) Tony commented that one of the rings looked like *Game of Thrones* because it resembled a serpent. In total, we spent about five minutes there.

As we were trying to decide whether to go to the Mexican restaurant across the street or keep looking, the kid from the jewelry store ran up behind us.

"You need to come with me," he said. "I need to talk to you about something."

"What do you need to talk to us about?" I said.

"Can you tell us what's going on?" Tony said.

The kid's eyes were very dark and frightening. He pointed at me. "You," he said. "I need to talk with *you*."

I refused to go back to the shop. I was certain he was going to pull out a gun, rob us, steal our passports, or make us pay him off.

He accused me of stealing a ring. He said he had video footage.

I hadn't. In the past, I'd definitely stolen the occasional lipstick, but those days were behind me. Thank god. But I was wearing a black raincoat with pockets that I frequently put my hands in and was worried he had a video of it looking like I'd stolen something.

Tony went into the shop, and I yelled at him to get out. The kid kept telling Tony to sit down. He had the landline cordless phone in his hands and said he was going to call the cops.

"Please do," I said. "I didn't steal anything. Call the cops. We're going to dinner." I was in a *fuck you* mood.

We walked across the street to the Mexican restaurant, our dinner decision made for us. We didn't want to run or go far because I thought it would make us seem guilty.

We ordered two margaritas and tacos. We let the manager know what was going on. He went across the street to the jewelry store, and when he came back, he said, "Just so you know, he is calling the cops."

"It's fine," I kept telling Tony. "They can't do anything,"

"We don't know what cops are like here," he said.

"True."

The two girls next to us asked what was going on and we told them. They were smoking cigarettes. Nonchalantly, they shook their heads and said nothing could be done without evidence.

Two sips into our margaritas, a Land Rover appeared. Three cops in army uniforms and lace-up boots called us over. I assumed they were going to talk to us. When I walked over, they asked me to return to my table and get my wallet and coat. Still naive, I figured they were going to search my stuff, but instead they took my license, Tony's passport, and handcuffed both of us.

I can't believe I've made it this long in my life without ever being handcuffed, I thought. (Tony had, twice.)

They ushered us into the back of the Land Rover. A machine gun in the front seat was pointing toward us. We asked what was going on, and the response was, "No English."

I felt calm; I was so relieved the kid at the jewelry store hadn't held us up at gunpoint. I was also in my element. I won't go so far as to say what many people do—that they thrive in chaos. It's just that fight-or-flight kicked in.

That said, we didn't know: if we'd been arrested, if we were going to jail, how far the police station was.

"You are accused of theft," one of the cops finally said, before he broke into song, some French a cappella.

The police station was only five minutes away from the restaurant. They took us into the station and removed the handcuffs, brought us to a room upstairs. The room had a desk, a few chairs, a bunk bed, and a TV. *Arabs Got Talent* was on.

Tony and I craned our necks to watch it for a while. There was nothing else to do. I looked around. There was a bright-blue

bag on a shelf that read DYNAMIC KIDS, and I thought these
guys couldn't be too bad, if they were shopping at a store like
that.

Tony leaned toward me and said, "You gotta admit, this is
worse than the tour."

"I'm not so sure I agree," I said.

I'd been thinking just the opposite. On the tour, I'd felt
lethargic, bored, irritable, impatient. Now I felt alert, high-energy, and curious.

Cigarette smoke swirled all over us, into our eyes and hair
and clothes. We couldn't use our phones to text anyone or google our rights, because neither of us had a data plan.

Another dude came in with a cup of coffee in one hand and
a cigarette in the other. His eyes were wide, and he was wearing
a sk8er-type sweatshirt. Tony told him he liked his sweatshirt.
At this point there were six men in the room with us.

"Is there Wi-Fi in here?" Tony asked. He was met with no
response except some snickering.

After about twenty-five minutes, it felt like we were watching the Three Stooges, but with Lebanese cops. It was just another day of work for all of them, and they had the rapport
and familiarity of a group of men who'd worked together for
a decade. The chubby one hid the short guy's phone. The bald
one with kind eyes FaceTimed with what sounded like his wife
and kids. He rarely spoke but when he smiled, it lit up the police station. He made a lot of eye contact with me. With Tony,

too. I couldn't tell if he felt compassion for us or just thought we were really dumb. Another cop, the one who'd sat in the back seat with us and sang in French, had the straightest nose I'd ever seen.

My favorite one was the chubby one, even though he was the most frightening. He had intense brown eyes and thick black hair. When he was funny, he was *really* funny, and when he was mean, it seemed he would kill someone with no remorse.

One of the cops got tired of *Arabs Got Talent* and changed the channel to the film *Platoon*.

They looked over at us.

"Ça va?"

"Oui." We shrugged, as if we had a choice, as if we could have said, "Actually I'd prefer a sitcom or a drama, maybe some comforting cartoons instead of watching people murder each other."

Enter another cop, who was apparently so tired he dramatically flopped down on the bottom bunk bed where my coat and scarf were. He pulled them over him as blankets. Slapstick. We all laughed.

One of them handed us our bill from the restaurant. They'd sent our bill—my fish tacos, Tony's chicken tacos, and two margaritas—to the station, after we didn't touch our food and they saw us get handcuffed.

"They want us to pay this?" Tony asked, and handed over his credit card.

"Nah," the cop grumbled and discarded it.

More men, more smoke. One man, not in a military uniform but in regular clothes, pulled up a chair near me and went on Facebook. I looked over his shoulder as he scrolled past what looked like memes about Jesus. One of the cops began sneaking selfies with the sleeping cop.

Someone brought in a printed photo of four rings. The printing was blurry and unclear. The top corner ring was the one I "stole." It was yellow gold and $550. All the rings I'd seen in the shop were silver.

A few of the cops took Tony out of the room. I had to pee so badly and I was playing a game with myself to see how long I could hold it because I didn't want to go through the trouble of asking to go. I realized I was thinking more about my having to pee than whatever was going on with Tony. I decided to send him positive vibes of love and safety. One of the cops who reminded me of Luigi from *Super Mario Bros.* opened a big bottle of Nestlé water, drank from it, handed it to someone else, and then wordlessly handed it to me. I thought this was sweet. I took what I could get. It had to be a good sign that we were all sharing a bottle of water.

When Tony walked back into the room, he had his jacket over his shoulder, his hair was messed up, and his face flushed.

"Did you get searched?"

"Yup," he said, annoyed. "Completely strip-searched and four squats. They laughed at me and told me all Americans look the same. They're calling in a female cop for you."

We waited for almost another hour for her to arrive. "La fille! La fille!" I kept hearing them say, looking at me.

Occasionally Tony and I would touch each other's legs or hold hands. It felt in some ways as if we were on drugs: senses heightened, slight perspiration on the forehead, going on adrenaline. After being apart for eight weeks, I felt happy we were stuck here together. For once, no obligations.

Tony realized he had the phone number for Michel, the sweet and friendly dude who owned and ran our hostel. We were not allowed to use a phone, so one of the cops did so for us. Michel answered the phone and showed up fifteen minutes later.

"This is completely unacceptable, what they've done to you," he said. "They cannot do this on no evidence."

Michel and the Luigi cop began yelling in Arabic, aggressively gesticulating. We watched, our heads going back and forth like kittens watching a string.

Finally, I was called into another room. The men stood outside the door as I went inside with a female cop. She took me into the corner and had me take everything off. She mimicked how to do a squat thrust. I did it, happy to get some exercise. I had a wedding coming up, after all. She went behind me and searched my hair. Had I ever been this intimate with a woman? Even when I change in front of my mom now, I turn my back.

I was terrified that Andreas, the kid working at the jewelry store, had planted the ring on me. As she slammed my clog boots on the cold, hard floor, I prayed to god a ring wouldn't fall out. It didn't. The men outside the room kept slamming on the door yelling words I couldn't understand, and the cop yelled back at them.

I asked her if I could use the bathroom. She nodded and waited outside the door. Though the toilet paper was nothing to write home about and I didn't have any underwear on, and people outside the doors were waiting for me, it was one of the best and most relaxing pees of my life.

"What would you do if I actually had the ring and put it on the desk right now?" I asked Tony.

He shook his head. "Too soon."

Because of my skin color (white) and my hair color (blond) I assumed that if I told someone I didn't steal a ring, they'd have to believe me. What if I were an Egyptian man? A Black teenager? What if my hair was short and I was with another woman? I didn't yet know about the Human Rights Watch report released in 2013 that reported that Lebanese police officials have threatened, beaten, and sometimes tortured gay, bisexual, and transgender people in their custody.

They took us down the hall.

"Where are we going?" Tony asked to no response.

We were brought into a room with a couple chairs and a desk. And—plot twist!—there was Andreas himself, sitting in one of the chairs.

They made me sit in a chair next to him, though I didn't want to. I didn't want to look at him.

Tony sat near the cop with the straight nose.

Andreas and Straight Nose started a conversation that got more heated every second. Michel came in and translated little snippets for Tony and me.

"He's saying he didn't actually see you steal the ring," Michel told me.

"Then why did he say he did? And that he had a video?"

"We don't know."

They took Andreas to get strip-searched in the back.

Now that I was officially unaccused, I could really sit back and enjoy the show.

Antoine, the owner of the jewelry store, came in, smoking, and sat with us. He looked at one of the rings I wear stacked on my fingers, and said he'd made a ring very similar to one of them many years ago. I asked if his wife ever asked him to make her rings and he responded, "Every second day." He told us the story of a bracelet he was wearing—he'd made it in the eighties and hasn't taken it off since. He wasn't wearing a wedding ring though he mentioned his wife often, like the time she washed his passport and he was detained because customs couldn't make out what it said.

Tony caught my eye and gestured to help him speed this interrogation process up. Maybe I was talking too much. I was excitable and caught up in the whole mystery. I couldn't figure it out, and I *love* figuring things out.

Why would Andreas say he saw me steal the ring if he didn't? Did he actually steal the ring to sell for money? But why would he call the cops if he stole the ring? Unless he had called the cops not thinking things would go this far. Maybe he didn't think he would also be called into the station as well. He could be friends with one of the cops. Or perhaps he gave the ring to the cops and just paid them off. Was he a drug addict and did he need the money for heroin? If he was trying to scare us and get us to give him money, why didn't he just threaten to call the cops and make us pay off the ring?

Maybe the ring was stolen by someone else earlier in the day, and he needed someone to blame. Either that, or he was evil and framing me.

The electricity went out. After a beat of silence, Antoine said, deadpan, "Welcome to Lebanon," and Tony and I burst out laughing.

Straight Nose found out Tony was a musician and perked up.

"You know Michael Jackson?" he said.

"He's great," I answered.

"He isn't great. He's—how do you say—super! My English isn't very good."

"Your English is better than my Arabic," Tony said, and we all laughed again. Straight Nose patted Tony's arm. He asked us if we wanted coffee, which of course we did. We were all old friends now.

Straight Nose made a phone call for the coffee. "Whitney's good," he said. He told us he sang in a band when he was younger, and I remembered him singing in the Land Rover when they'd picked us up hours earlier.

The coffee was espresso in little brown cups that said LIVE LOVE on them. There was a hefty amount of sugar on the bottom, which I scraped out and ate with my finger.

Michel and Antoine were in a heated discussion (in English) about Antoine getting cameras for his store. Michel was for it; Antoine said he never would. Michel was telling him how stupid that was. Antoine was saying he didn't like the feeling of cameras in the store. Michel said, then things like this will happen. Antoine said, yes, this is the third time something similar has happened. Michel said, that's why you need cameras.

Tony gave his account of the night. I gave my account of the night. Everything was written down by hand.

They got me my coat and scarf and we headed downstairs. We were getting out! They half-heartedly shook our hands and said, "Sorry."

✦

The perfect ring ended up being closer than I thought. At home, there was a ring my dad had given my mom for one of their anniversaries and I'd forever called it "my mom's emerald ring" and been in love with it as a kid. Since we didn't own any expensive things, shopped at Sears, JCPenney, and Filene's Basement, I coveted it. My mom kept it in a jewelry box with my baby teeth. Finally, in my late twenties, she gifted it to me, and then it lay around in my jewelry box because it was too big for me. Sadie liked to try it on and to wonder aloud how much it was worth. She liked to say that it fit her, as kids do when they try on their parents' high heels.

Looking at it when I returned home from Lebanon, I decided to get it resized.

When I brought it into the jewelry store and it was cleaned, I learned the stone wasn't green, and it wasn't emerald. It was blue topaz.

"It's a good thing that it isn't emerald, actually," the woman at the jewelry store told me. "Emerald breaks and cracks easily."

I was glad the ring wasn't a so-called weak emerald, because getting handcuffed together a mere month before our wedding—never blaming each other, not once bickering, managing to make it a memorable, loving learning experience—showed me something about my relationship. It was the opposite of fragile.

On the plane from Beirut to Doha, Qatar, where we'd have an eight-hour layover, I turned to Tony.

"What would you do if I just silently pulled the ring out and put it on your tray table?"

"We'd have *a lot* of talking to do," he responded, and we laughed our asses off.

At the Doha international airport, we walked by what looked like sleeping lounges, though there were two different rooms, one for men and one for women. Though we were forced to separate, neither of us had felt more together.

BLENDED FAMILY

Being a stepmom has some undertones of what being queer feels like: they can both be invisible. They are both behind-the-scenes. People can't tell from looking at you. They can also look at you and make an assumption of what you are.

In her book of microessays, *No Relation*, Paula Carter calls herself an "almost-mother." In a *New York Times* article, she writes about not having a name for the relationship she had with a long-term partner's children: "I was not the boys' mother—they had one of those; I was not even their step-mother. But, I was something. When you realize you are out-side of what has been deemed normal, what has been named and defined, these are the things you feel you lack: Dignity, autonomy, belonging. And a shared understanding of the role you play."

Biological mothers like to say you don't know what having a baby is like until you have one. What is said less often is that biological moms don't know what having a stepkid overnight is like, either.

The mark of motherhood has been well-documented; the mark of stepmotherhood less so.

In *The Birth of an Adoptive, Foster or Stepmother*, Barbara Waterman writes: "Although I did recite a Zuni adoption prayer to my daughters during the wedding ceremony to their father, the enormity of my life change remained hidden without social rituals to mark it publicly."

Stepmom contains two opposite ideas: it epitomizes blurred lines, gray areas: you're not a mom and you're not *not* a mom. But it's also a label.

In her memoir, *Stepmother*, Marianne Lile writes, "In a not-so-subtle way, it does conjure up a loss: death or divorce. Either way, it points to the demise of a relationship along the way. And now I had this label attached to me. What happens when you take on a label?"

✦

The first time Sadie said "I love you" to me is as vivid as any time a partner did—if not more so. It was March and she was leaving for D.C. Tony and I had been together for almost one year, and we weren't living together or engaged yet.

Tony left the apartment to start the car but Sadie hung back in the stairwell and said "I love you" very quietly.

"What?" I asked, and she sheepishly said it again, but looked me in the eye.

"I love you, too," I said.

My friend Emma, who is dating a man with a four-year-old boy, said her heart raced as she was singing the song "Skinnamarink" with him and she realized as they led up to the chorus, that they would be saying "I love you" for the first time.

People throw around the term "chosen family" for their friends. According to *The SAGE Encyclopedia of Marriage, Family, and Couples Counseling*, "Chosen families are nonbiological kinship bonds, whether legally recognized or not, deliberately chosen for the purpose of mutual support and love." The term originated within the LGBTQ community and was used to describe early queer gatherings like the Harlem drag balls of the late nineteenth century.

Aren't stepkids your chosen family, though? Aren't you *choosing* to marry a partner who has kids?

✦

On Christmases, the blendedness of blended families is exposed, becomes high-definition. Sadie usually spends the first half the day with her mom and the rest with us. I spend half the day with my dad and the rest with my mom. This means Sadie goes from her mom's house to her dad's house to *my* dad's house to my mom's house. That's a lot of houses. It is passed off to kids as, "You get two Christmases! More presents!"

Kids love Christmas, and I am not implying the movement on Christmas Day is a negative thing. It's just something people whose parents are together and wake up and stay in one house all day and go to sleep at that same house at night will not experience. The packing of the bags, change in surroundings, shuffling of presents.

In 2020, Sadie and I sat together as we watched our friends JD and Marty get married. Marty had a ten-year-old child, Willow, from a previous marriage. JD, whom Willow clearly adored, was going to be their stepdad. We had dinner with them regularly, and the kids became close through a shared love of Harry Potter, playing Clue, and lemonade stands in the summer.

Now, at the wedding, JD read vows to Willow: "The first time I met you, you were hiding behind a door, trying not to be seen but wanting to see. I knew you were scared but I also knew you were courageous. I knew that your life was already chaotic. You move between homes. You move between people. You move between men.

"I promise you patience, unwavering support and love, for you, for your dad, our chosen family. And I choose you Willow. I *choose* you. No matter what you come to believe in this world, no matter what mistakes you will make, I choose you."

Willow, normally sassy, a little guarded, choked back tears and placed their hand over their heart.

✦

Spalding Gray referred to himself as his stepdaughter Marissa's "accidental dad." Gray's slim memoir *Morning, Noon and Night* chronicles his blended family with two biological sons and his eleven-year-old stepdaughter, Marissa, who he says was "like a strange mirror to me." In a scene where Gray's wife is pumping gas, he writes: "Marissa, sure that the smell would cause her brain cells to die, rode with her head out the window for an hour. She will survive and thrive. There is no doubt in my mind about that."

On the ten-year anniversary of Gray's suicide in 2004, NPR interviewed his wife and Marissa, whom they called his daughter:

"He taught me how to think, how to see the world," Marissa said. "And I was reading one of Spalding's books and he wrote, 'I know Marissa will survive and thrive for her whole life.' And that's such a gift, to have a parent write down how they feel about you."

I have finally learned to cook because I like feeding my boyfriend and daughter. Is she my daughter? I make her oatmeal and stuffed peppers; she loves sweet-potato-and-farro bowls. I put cheese on everything so she'll eat more of it; she has Wisconsin Dairyland in her blood. She gives me a thumbs-up and scarfs it down. Even when she was six, she'd ask for a million toppings on her pizza at restaurants: olives, anchovies, peppers, pepperoni, onion, and sausage. "I wasn't expecting that," one waiter said, impressed by her palate.

Before I could even imagine marrying or being a mom or stepmom, my favorite films were the ones with "out-of-bounds" relationships. In *My Girl*, the character Vada becomes close with the woman who works in her house. In *Stepmom*, Jena Malone and Julia Roberts and finally bond while driving in the car, passing lipstick back and forth and singing along to "Ain't No Mountain High Enough." In *Corrina, Corrina*, the nanny, Corrina, is the only person that Molly, whose mom has just passed away, will communicate with, which she does by tapping her nose once for no and twice for yes. I have shown Sadie all these movies, which she loved.

"I choose things that I had once loved," Paula Carter writes. "That is one of the privileges of caring for children."

I tell her things no one ever told me: that fighting can be okay so long as there is resolution and respect. That just because Tony and I had a fight doesn't mean we will break up. Wearing new boots on your first day of school is good luck. That the reason I am in bed during a sun-sweat day is because an egg is traveling through me.

Is that what tampons are for? she asks. I don't like having cramps, I've had them swimming, she says. So a pad is like a diaper, so twelve-year-olds kind of have to walk around wearing a diaper? Are the tampons because otherwise the blood will go everywhere?

In *The Argonauts*, Maggie Nelson writes: "Every time I see the word *stepchild* in an obituary, as in 'X is survived by three

children and two stepchildren,' or whenever an adult acquaintance says something like, 'Oh, sorry, I can't make it—I'm visiting my stepdad this weekend,' or when, during the Olympics,
the camera pans the audience and the voiceover says, 'there's
X's stepmother, cheering him on,' my heart skips a beat, just to
hear the sound of the bond made public, made positive."

On Thursdays I picked Sadie up from school at 3:30. At
3:00 p.m. I left the apartment to find a taco truck in front of
our driveway, blocking the car. I panicked, already running a
few minutes late.

"You're blocking my driveway," I told the man behind the
counter. He just stared at me, and I added, "And I have to go
pick up my kid."

My kid. It was the first time uttering these words. The
power to them. How quickly he moved the truck. How hard I
hit the gas pedal to get to the school on time.

My kid . . .

My kid. My kid. My kid.

✦

In her essay "In the Shadow of a Fairy Tale," Leslie Jamison
has an epic tribute to being a stepparent, a role she stepped
into through death, not divorce. It was in Jamison's article I
learned about the Icelandic folktale "The Good Stepmother."

Apparently, the tale is so rare, only three versions have been collected in Norway, Turkey, and Croatia.

The King's wife, the Queen, dies, and the King says he will not marry again because stepmothers are mean, and he doesn't want his daughter to suffer. He still falls in love with Hildur, but she won't marry him unless he lets her live alone with his daughter for three years before the wedding.

In Jamison's words: "Their marriage is made possible by her willingness to invest in a relationship with his daughter that exists apart from him, as its own fierce flame."

"You are the best version of yourself as a stepmom," my mom said.

✦

When Kamala Harris was nominated a vice presidential candidate in August 2020, her sister, niece, and stepdaughter created a video telling the world about family life with Kamala. "You're a rock," her sister says, "not just for our dad but for three generations of our big, blended family."

"How do you *love like a rock*?" My mom told me Sadie asked her this in the car, when she heard Paul Simon's "Loves Me Like a Rock" on the radio.

"How do you *adopt a highway*?" Sadie asked me, seeing a sign, reminding me of the days I'd drive around and see the foster parent signs. I only see them occasionally these days. I suppose they're seasonal.

✦

At his wedding, my friend JD kept repeating, "because I choose you," to Willow. Sadie took my hand. I cried; she smiled. It was New Year's Eve. Dozens of candles were lit, tracing the inside of the church. Sadie and I were sitting alone, as Tony was playing piano softly underneath the vows.

"I choose you," I whispered to Sadie. It seemed like the thing to say at the moment. And I meant it.

"I choose *you*," she whispered back, and squeezed.

THINGS THAT HELPED II

There were a few consecutive birthdays where my friend Fran set up tarot readings for me with her psychic medium, Kaylene, in Portland, Oregon. The previous two years, I'd done the sessions over the phone, but in May 2017, I had a reading to do at Marylhurst University in Oregon, so I would be staying in Portland for a week visiting friends.

I drove to Kaylene's in the sun. She wore all black and we sat at her little kitchen table. I recorded the session on my phone.

I'd just turned thirty-one and met Tony and Sadie. I didn't know anything about PMDD, but I knew stuff was coming up from falling in love so quickly. I knew I felt psycho.

I didn't listen to the recording again until 2021.

The first card she pulled was the Ten of Pentacles, reversed. She said it represented disharmony within the family. "Falling out of grace. The family tree does not have solid roots. It can mean depriving energy. The feeling of *I don't have enough.* Where are my resources? Where is my community?" She said it represented generations: parents, grandparents, heritage.

"The older I get," I heard myself say on the recording, "the more my family feels split, splintered."

Kaylene said, "Your heart is really talking to me. I'm probably going to tear up. I think your heart realizes he has total unconditional love for you. You don't have to pretend your family was anything better than it was. And Tony's fine with that." Her voice cracks.

Kaylene said, "That's going to be something that's going to take you a while to be able to receive. For so long you let this run your patterns in relationships."

I said, "It's amazing to think I have a chance to have a family that's whole."

I said, "I always said I wouldn't get married until I knew I wouldn't get divorced."

I told Kaylene that when Tony said, "I'd marry you in a heartbeat," it made me want to run from the table.

Kaylene said, "He is just as flawed and broken as you are."

The next card Kaylene pulled was the Two of Cups.

Kaylene said, "This card is saying: Let's do this. I'm willing to risk my heart. It is mutual. Both people come with the same amount in their cups. Everything he has to offer you, you have to offer him, too, even if it is in totally different ways. The cup represents the heart."

She pulled the Two of Swords next.

Kaylene said, "You're going to great lengths to try to protect your heart. Are you willing to kill the story that goes *I can't be in a relationship unless I know I won't get hurt?* Are you willing to get married even if you don't know if you're going to get divorced?"

"Uck. It's hard for me," I said. "It's really hard for me. It is really hard to let that go."

Kaylene said, "Bring love to it. Bring gold, bring rose, bring honey. You're powerless over those thoughts and over your little brain saying *you're going to get hurt.* Surrender!"

Kaylene said, "The heart and the brain are very connected and now your heart, having been hurt, is wired that way."

Kaylene said, "Admit your powerlessness and turn it over to the Goddess."

Kaylene said, "When something is patterned in the brain, that's something really hard to fix with our will alone."

Kaylene said, "What are your shields? Do you need all your shields or can you let some go?"

I told Kaylene that in the past I'd always purposely sought out doomed relationships. That I sought out triangulations.

Kaylene said to create a new kind of triangle: the love of Goddess, then the love of self, then the beloved. That's the new triangle, the healthy triangle, she said.

Kaylene said I had healing to do. That I was guarded, pent up. That I needed to envision my brain and mind and head blossoming like a flower. She told me I had to heal the generations before me. It would be hard work, she said.

Kaylene said, "Give up duality. Give your brain a break.

You're trying to do the Goddess's job. Let the Goddess do that! Stop trying to predict the future."

Kaylene said, "If you can do the work of dissolving and healing, that will ripple through the bloodline."

Kaylene said, "When you were a kid, using a shield was a good idea. But as you grew it kept negative thoughts in, and is keeping out the divine. Let divine love in through the crown chakra. Let in the sunlight, starlight, moonlight, the celestial."

When I left, the sun enveloped me. I sat on the sidewalk and called Tony. I was surprised he answered. I was still surprised by someone being available to me, answering on the first ring.

THINGS THAT HELPED III

Thylox Bar Soap from the Grandpa Soap Company

Renée Rouleau Anti Bump Solution (formerly known as Anti Cyst Treatment)

Walgreens Acne Spot Drying Lotion

Eva Naturals Vitamin C Plus Skin Clearing Serum

Niacinamide

Lactic acid

Glycolic acid

Salicylic acid

THE CEREMONY

"*Every* period is an *irregular* period," comedian Michelle Wolf is known for saying. "It's not like a paycheck where it arrives on the same day every month. Your period is more like an outdoor cat—you know it's gonna come back at some point but you're never positive when, and you have *no idea* what it's gonna have in its mouth."

I don't have that irregularity; I can set my watch to my period. Day 28, in the morning, every (goddamn) month. As much as I'd tried to manipulate it, I was due to be on day 2 of my period on my wedding day.

When I went to acupuncture recently and was asked about my cycle, I told him it was much better than the last time I'd seen him a year earlier, that I'd shrunk and healed the symptoms through lifestyle: diet, supplements, Prozac, exercise, therapy. He seemed pleased, proud, even.

"People think they have to live that way," he said. "Uncomfortable and suffering. But they don't."

"Yeah," I responded, conflicted, thoughtful, and sort of moved by his statement.

Another acupuncturist who specializes in the menstrual cycle, Talia Brooks-Salzman, told me: "Blood houses the heart and allows us to feel protected and safe. If we lose too much blood during menses, we are much more vulnerable to the outside world."

♦

We were married late May in my mom's backyard at the house I grew up in; we were married in the backyard of the house where my mom was remarried, the backyard of the house where my parents were divorced. ("It's a big deal to make a sentence." —Lidia Yuknavitch) The spring forsythias were blazing yellow, in bloom, reaching, and I wore my Thinx period underwear under my non-white dress. At the reception, I'd put a basket filled with tampons and pads and ibuprofen for my guests, but also for me.

We'd had some fights over the wedding playlist. I felt he was hogging it. While we were arguing, Tony said my voice sounded like nails on a chalkboard. His comment made my voice go up another octave. He was on his way to do laundry and return a werewolf mask he'd gotten at Party City. He often bought and returned costumes to use for piano ragtime videos. So while we were screaming at each other and he was trying to leave the apartment, he kept setting down, then picking back up, the werewolf mask. We finally couldn't ignore how funny it was. After he left, I did the dishes as a peace offering. I napped, to hopefully sleep off some PMDD, and then I texted him, "If you wanted to pick cookies or brownies or something I wouldn't be mad." He returned with a bag of four perfect chocolate brownies from the health food store. I thought maybe this could be a new tool: ask for something that I need that he can actually do (not ephemeral things like, *Support me! Be nice to me!*). It works because I get something I want (brownies) and he gets to feel like he did something "right" and it gives him something tangible to do. Plus, he gets brownies, too.

Instead of looking at my period as a hurdle on my wedding day, I decided to see it as an ally. I decided to be the person who honored her period. Felt the strength and empowerment in it. Ah, here you are. Of course you are with me. Integrated, finally. Finally integrated.

Put your arm around it.

Heal your inner child and all that stuff, Google it.

Some girls have a little less pep.

This cyclical behavior can break even the deepest of bonds.

Whatever they're experiencing, they're experiencing.

Did you forget?

I thought about a quote from *The Diary of a Young Girl*, where Anne Frank writes: "Whenever I get my period (and that's only been three times), I have the feeling that in spite of all the pain, discomfort and mess, I'm carrying around a sweet secret. So even though it's a nuisance, in a certain way I'm always looking forward to the time when I'll feel that secret inside me once again."

And on our honeymoon that fall—though I knew it was probably coming, a combination of a sixth sense and my period app—I began bleeding the moment our plane touched down in Lisbon, Portugal. My period was with me on my wedding day and on my honeymoon. I woke up with it on my thirty-third birthday and my thirty-fourth birthday. This is not for dramatic effect, and it's not a literary device. These are just facts. It's me and my shadow, my teacher; the natural plot of my existence.

Acknowledgments

My editor, Yuka Igarashi: Thank you for your developmental and line editing, your collaboration, your vision. Thank you for getting this book in ways I didn't yet get it. You are a true listener. I enjoyed every second of working together, and am deeply grateful for everything you did to make this book happen. Every time I have my period now, I will think of you. <3

Thank you, Carole Maso, for being the first reader, your belief in me, and actionable feedback. You changed the way I think about writing.

Thank you, Becky Sternal, for supporting me in PMDD and otherwise.

Thank you, Sarah Lyn Rogers, for your communication, intelligent notes, and thoughtfulness.

Thank you, Michael Salu, for so many cover designs I loved, it was hard to choose just one.

Thank you to everyone on the Soft Skull team, especially: Megan Fishmann, Rachel Fershleiser, Lena Moses-Schmitt, Wah-Ming Chang, and Jordan Koluch.

Thank you to editors Jess Grose, Sari Botton, Shannon Keating, Elizabeth Ellen, and Kristin Iversen for publishing variations of these chapters in *Lenny Letter*, *Longreads*, *Buzz-Feed*, *Hobart*, and *NYLON*.

Thank you, LK: reading and talking about books and plot and writers with you is the privilege of my life. Thank you for your humor, kindness, your passion for bookstores and the written word. Thanks for sharing your library with me.

Thank you, JD Urban and Marty Geren, for your sweet friendship, and countless family dinners.

Thank you to my extended family, including my aunts, cousins, students, friends of friends for sharing your personal period stories with me for "The Linen Closet."

Thank you to the International Association For Premenstrual Disorders, especially Amanda LaFleur, Sandi McDonald, and Brett Buchert.

Spruceton Inn, specifically Casey Scieszka: thank you for the time and space to write.

My gratitude to The Cabins Residency and Courtney Maum, Sebastian Barreveld, and Antje Barreveld for the time and space to write in Lincoln, Massachusetts.

Thank you, Mom: you are so lit.

Thank you, Dad: for your hurdy-gurdy tampon anecdote.

TK: Thank you for supporting the hotel writing binges, the do-not-disturb sign, learning about PMDD with me, and teaching me what real love could look like. Thank you for your humor and grace. Marry me!

Thank you, Karina: in 2017 you told me you wanted to hear more about this red zone I kept referencing.

Resources

PMS/PMDD Support Links

International Association for Premenstrual Disorders: iapmd
.org

Reddit: reddit.com/r/PMDD

PMS Forum: www.pms.org.uk

Natalie Ryan Hebert: natalieryanhebert.com/the-red-tent

Period Girl: nicolejardim.com

Books That Helped

WomanCode by Alisa Vitti

*Moody Bitches: The Truth About the Drugs You're Taking, the
Sleep You're Missing, the Sex You're Not Having, and What's
Really Making You Crazy* by Julie Holland, MD

Anger by Thich Nhat Hanh

A Mind of Your Own by Kelly Brogan, MD

The Female Brain by Louann Brizendine, MD

*We Need to Talk About PMDD: Living with Premenstrual Dys-
phoric Disorder* by Sara McGinnis

The PMDD Phenomenon by Diana L. Dell and Carol Svec

It Didn't Start with You by Mark Wolynn

The Body Keeps the Score by Bessel van der Kolk, MD

Transforming Relationships by Donna R. Baker-Gilroy, PsyD, and David R. Gilroy, PsyD

CHLOE CALDWELL is the author of three books: *I'll Tell You in Person*, *Women*, and *Legs Get Led Astray*. Her essays have been published in *The New York Times*, *Bon Appétit*, *The Cut*, *The Strategist*, *BuzzFeed*, *NYLON*, *VICE*, *Longreads*, and many anthologies. Her essay "Hungry Ghost" was listed as Notable in *The Best American Nonrequired Reading 2017*. She lives in Hudson, New York, and teaches creative writing online at Writing Workshops, LitReactor, and the Fine Arts Work Center. Find out more at www.chloesimonne.com.